Urology Pearls

MARTIN I. RESNICK, MD
Lester Persky Professor and Chairman
Department of Urology
Case Western Reserve University School of Medicine
Cleveland, Ohio

ANTHONY J. SCHAEFFER, MD
Herman L. Kretschmer Professor and Chairman
Department of Urology
Northwestern University Medical School
Chicago, Illinois

Series Editors

STEVEN A. SAHN, MD
Professor of Medicine and Director
Division of Pulmonary and
 Critical Care Medicine
Medical University of South Carolina
Charleston, South Carolina

JOHN E. HEFFNER, MD
Professor and Vice Chairman
Department of Medicine
Medical University of South Carolina
Charleston, South Carolina

HANLEY & BELFUS, INC. / Philadelphia

Publisher: HANLEY & BELFUS, INC.
              Medical Publishers
              210 S. 13th Street
              Philadelphia, PA 19107
              (215) 546-7293, 800-962-1892
              FAX (215) 790-9330
              Website: http://www.hanleyandbelfus.com

Library of Congress Cataloging-in-Publication Data

Urology pearls / edited by Martin I. Resnick, Anthony J. Schaeffer.
        p.   cm.—(The Pearls Series®)
     Includes bibliographical references and index.
     ISBN 1-56053-351-X (alk. paper)
     1. Urology Case studies.   2. Genitourinary organs—Diseases
Case studies.   I. Resnick, Martin I.   II. Schaeffer, Anthony J.
     [DNLM: 1. Urologic Diseases—diagnosis Case Report.
2. Urologic Diseases—diagnosis Problems and Exercises.
3. Urologic Diseases—therapy Case Report.   4. Urologic Diseases—
therapy Problems and Exercises.   WJ 18.2 U7778 1999]
RC872.U715   2000
616.6'09—DC21
DNLM/DLC
for Library of Congress   99-32134
                                                                  CIP

UROLOGY PEARLS   ISBN 1-56053-351-X

Last digit is the print number: 9 8 7 6 5 4 3 2 1

CONTENTS

Patient   **Page**

CONTRIBUTORS

Andrew Altman, MD
Resident, Department of Urology, Case Western Reserve University School of Medicine, Cleveland, Ohio

Ahmad Bafa, MD
Resident, Department of Urology, Case Western Reserve University School of Medicine, Cleveland, Ohio

Robert A. Batler, MD
Resident, Department of Urology, Northwestern University Medical School, Chicago, Illinois

Lynn W. Blunt, Jr., MD
Resident, Department of Urology, Northwestern University Medical School, Chicago, Illinois

Donald R. Bodner, MD
Professor, Department of Urology, Case Western Reserve University School of Medicine, Cleveland, Ohio

Robert E. Brannigan, MD
Assistant Professor, Department of Urology, Northwestern University Medical School, Chicago, Illinois

Scott L. Brown, MD
Chief Resident, Department of Urology, Case Western Reserve University School of Medicine, Cleveland, Ohio

Bruce I. Carlin, MD
Resident, Department of Urology, Northwestern University Medical School, Chicago, Illinois

J. Quentin Clemens, MD
Resident, Department of Urology, Northwestern University Medical School, Chicago, Illinois

Evan Cohn, MD
Clinical Instructor, Department of Surgery, University of Pittsburgh, Pittsburgh, Pennsylvania

Jack S. Elder, MD
Professor of Urology and Pediatrics, Case Western Reserve University School of Medicine, Cleveland; Director of Pediatric Urology, Rainbow Babies' and Children's Hospital, Cleveland, Ohio

Jason D. Engel, MD
Clinical Assistant Professor, Department of Urology, George Washington University Hospital, Washington, District of Columbia

Chris H. Gonzalez, MD
Chief Resident, Department of Urology, Northwestern University Medical School, Chicago, Illinois

Christopher A. Haas, MD
Assistant Professor, Department of Urology, Case Western Reserve University School of Medicine, Cleveland, Ohio

John Chance Hairston, MD
Resident, Department of Urology, Northwestern University Medical School, Chicago, Illinois

Steven E. Kahan, MD, JD
Resident, Department of Urology, Case Western Reserve University School of Medicine, Cleveland, Ohio

Jason L. Kelly, MD
Resident, Department of Urology, Northwestern Memorial Hospital, Chicago, Illinois

Samuel C. Kim, MD
Resident, Department of Urology, Northwestern University Medical School, Chicago, Illinois

Mark E. Kolligian, MD
Assistant Clinical Professor, Department of Urology, New York Medical College, Valhalla, New York

H. Merrill Matschke, MD
Staff Physician, Department of Urology, Northwestern University Medical School, Chicago, Illinois

Michael L. Paik, MD
Resident, Department of Urology, Case Western Reserve University School of Medicine, Cleveland, Ohio

Rashmi Patel, MD
Chief Resident, Department of Urology, Case Western Reserve University School of Medicine, Cleveland, Ohio

Kent Perry, MD
Resident, Department of Urology, Northwestern University Medical School, Chicago, Illinois

Melissa D. Reigle, MD
Chief Resident, Department of Urology, Case Western Reserve University School of Medicine, Cleveland, Ohio

Martin I. Resnick, MD
Lester Persky Professor and Chairman, Department of Urology, Case Western Reserve University School of Medicine, Cleveland; Director, Department of Urology, University Hospitals of Cleveland, Cleveland, Ohio

Anthony J. Schaeffer, MD
Herman L. Kretschmer Professor and Chairman, Department of Urology, Northwestern University Medical School, Chicago, Illinois

Richard A. Schoor, MD
Chief Resident, Department of Urology, Northwestern University Medical School, Chicago, Illinois

Allen D. Seftel, MD
Associate Professor, Department of Urology, Case Western Reserve University School of Medicine, Cleveland, Ohio

Norm D. Smith, MD
Chief Resident, Department of Urology, Northwestern University Medical School, Chicago, Illinois

J. Patrick Spirnak, MD
Associate Professor, Department of Urology, Case Western Reserve University School of Medicine, Cleveland; Director of Urology, MetroHealth Medical Center, Cleveland, Ohio

Jeffrey A. Stern, MD, MPH
Resident, Department of Urology, Northwestern University Medical School, Chicago, Illinois

Aaron Sulman, MD
Resident, Department of Urology, Case Western Reserve University School of Medicine, Cleveland, Ohio

Herbert M. User, MD
Resident, Department of Urology, Northwestern Memorial Hospital, Chicago, Illinois

Ahmad Z. Vafa, MD
Chief Resident, Department of Urology, Case Western Reserve University School of Medicine, Cleveland, Ohio

John David Wegryn, MD
Resident, Department of Urology, Case Western Reserve University School of Medicine, Cleveland, Ohio

Adam C. Weiser, MD
Resident, Department of Urology, Northwestern University Medical School, Chicago, Illinois

FOREWORD

The thoughtful surgeon must master a broad array of skills in managing clinical problems. Successful surgical interventions depend on the surgeon's ability to accurately diagnose the patient's condition. Careful decision-making then matches the most appropriate intervention to the specific problem at hand. The intervention itself requires experience, skill, and knowledge to promote a successful technical outcome.

Considering these multiple challenges facing our surgery colleagues, we are delighted to extend The Pearls Series® for the first time to a surgical discipline. *Urology Pearls* challenges readers with a case-based clinical problem. The discussion that follows provides a cutting-edge review of the general topic as well as the unique aspects of the presented patient's condition. Especially important patient care considerations are captured at the end of the discussion as "Clinical Pearls." This format has assisted students and residents as they enter their medical career and experienced clinicians as they continue to hone their clinical skills.

We congratulate Drs. Resnick and Schaeffer for their successful presentation of a challenging series of case problems and insightful discussions from their clinical practice. They have captured superbly the goals of The Pearls Series®, which include stimulating readers toward life-long learning by observing their patients, by seeking answers to uncertain clinical problems, and by adding to their own list of clinical pearls as their experience grows.

John E. Heffner, MD
Steven A. Sahn, MD
SERIES EDITORS

PREFACE

Teaching by example is known to be effective, and *Urology Pearls* employs this principle to good effect by presenting case histories that emphasize various points in patient diagnosis and treatment. This book is one of a series that has been successful in educating medical students and house staff in particular specialties. *Urology Pearls* has maintained this tradition.

The patients described here typically are seen not only by physicians specializing in urology, but by primary care physicians as well. They demonstrate interesting but common urologic problems that require appropriate patient assessment before proper treatment can be initiated. For some cases, the "answer" is quite apparent, and the management of the patient is noncontroversial. Other cases are more complex, and after the initial presentation, various disorders must be excluded before the correct diagnosis is established and discussed. In a step-by-step manner, specific diseases are discarded, and the appropriateness of others becomes more evident.

It is anticipated that this text will be used by those learning the field and also by established professionals as a quick review on specific disorders. We hope that *Urology Pearls* will be as useful as the rest of The Pearls Series®.

The authors wish to acknowledge their associated faculty and residents who assisted in the development of this text. Additionally, we would like to acknowledge the assistance of Jacqueline M. Mahon and William J. Lamsback of Hanley & Belfus, Inc., who have been so supportive throughout this process.

Martin I. Resnick, MD
Anthony J. Schaeffer, MD

Dedication

Vicky, Andy, Jeff, Missy, and Katelin

&

Kathy, Christine, Ted, Anne, and Anthony

PATIENT 1

A 34-year-old woman with Cushing's syndrome

A 34-year-old woman presents with a 1-year history of progressive 50-pound weight gain, worsening acne, easy bruisability, frequent headaches, and emotional lability.

Physical Examination: Temperature 37°; pulse 75; blood pressure 180/90; respiration 30. General: truncal obesity; atrophic musculature. Skin: severe acne; multiple striae on torso.

Laboratory Findings: WBC 7600/μl, Hct 38%, platelets 297,000/μl. Na$^+$ 137 mEq/L, K$^+$ 4.0 mEq/L, Cl$^-$ 125 mEq/L. CO$_2$ 20 mmol/L. Bun 10 mg/dl, creatinine 0.8 mg/dl, serum glucose 257 mg/dl. Abdominal/pelvic computed tomography: 5-cm left adrenal mass; no calcifications or necrosis; atrophic right adrenal gland. 24-hour urine free cortisol: 100 μg (elevated).

Questions: What is the etiology of this patient's symptoms? How should this symptom complex be evaluated and treated?

Diagnosis: Adrenal cortical adenoma

Discussion: The patient's symptom complex is diagnostic of Cushing's syndrome, which results from excessive levels of circulating glucocorticoids produced by the zona fasciculata and zona reticularis of the adrenal cortex. This syndrome has multiple etiologies, and effective treatment depends upon identifying the cause.

Endogenous causes of Cushing's syndrome include Cushing's disease (resulting from pituitary hypersecretion of adrenocorticotropic hormone [ACTH]), adrenal adenomas, and adrenal carcinomas. Another cause is ectopic secretion of ACTH or corticotropic-releasing hormone (CRH) from metastatic tumors such as pulmonary oat cell, carcinoid, epithelial carcinoma of thymus, islet cell tumor of pancreas, thyroid carcinoma, and, rarely, pheochromocytoma.

Exogenous sources—for example, steroid-containing oral medications or creams/lotions—also must be ruled out as a possible cause. Exogenous sources are the most common cause of this syndrome.

To diagnose the etiology, Cushing's syndrome must first be documented by measuring two or three consecutive 24-hour urine free cortisol levels. If cortisol levels are elevated (indicative of the syndrome), a low-dose dexamethasone suppression test is then performed. Normal individuals typically are able to suppress cortisol levels to less than 2–5 µg/dl and 24-hour cortisol secretion to less than 20 µg.

Once Cushing's syndrome is verified, several diagnostic tests are done to identify the etiology. Plasma ACTH and cortisol are measured concurrently by two-site immunoradiometric assay. If cortisol is greater than 50 µg/dl and ACTH is less than 5 pg/ml, then the patient has a primary ACTH-independent adrenal Cushing's syndrome. Conversely, if the ACTH is greater than 50 pg/ml, then the patient has an ACTH-dependent process (Cushing's disease, or ectopic source of ACTH or CRH). A high-dose dexamethasone suppression test also can be done, checking plasma and urine cortisol levels. In cases of adrenal adenomas and carcinomas, cortisol secretion is *not* suppressed. With pituitary disease, a 50% or greater suppression of cortisol occurs. Petrosal venous sampling of ACTH also can be used to diagnose Cushing's disease.

In addition to differentiating primary adrenal causes from other etiologies of Cushing's syndrome, clinical and biological markers can be used to differentiate adrenal adenomas from carcinomas. Virilization in women and feminization in men tends to be indicative of adrenal carcinoma rather than adenoma. Also, elevated 17-ketosteroid, dehydroepiandrosterone sulfate, and lactate dehydrogenase levels are more common with carcinomas than adenomas. Both adrenal diseases are more common in women.

Radiographic studies also can be valuable diagnostic tools. Computed tomography (CT), magnetic resonance imaging (MRI), intravenous pyelography, NP-59 scintillation scans, arteriography, and venography can be useful. A CT scan allows diagnosis of adrenal masses with hyperplasia, demonstrating diffuse thickening and elongation of the adrenal rami and occasionally showing nodular cortical hyperplasia. Adrenal carcinomas, which for the most part have a poor prognosis, usually are greater than 6 centimeters in size and frequently show calcification and necrosis. MRI can differentiate adrenal cortical carcinomas from adenomas because the former are hypointense relative to the liver and spleen on T1-weighted images and hyperintense relative to the liver and spleen on T2-weighted images. Adenomas show no significant change in intensity when comparing T1- and T2-weighted images.

Since the etiologies of Cushing's syndrome vary widely, so do the treatments. The goals of treatment are: decrease daily cortisol secretion to normal, eradicate health-threatening tumors, avoid permanent endocrine deficiency, and avoid permanent medication dependence. With these goals in mind, both adrenal adenomas and adrenal carcinomas are treated with surgical removal, although adrenal cortical carcinomas have a 5-year survival rate of only 35%. Postoperatively, carcinoma patients are followed by hormonal markers and can be treated with mitotane or o,p'-DDD chemotherapy. Adrenal masses 5 centimeters or greater in size discovered incidentally or those showing an increase in size during regular followup also are removed.

Be aware that cushingoid patients are at increased operative risk because of their obesity, diabetes, osteopenia, and increased susceptibility to infection. It is beneficial to treat these patients preoperatively with metabolic blockers such as metyrapone to reverse some of their clinical abnormalities prior to surgery. Also, all patients require glucocorticoid replacement (i.e., hydrocortisone sodium succinate and cortisone acetate) throughout the surgical procedure and postoperatively until they recover contralateral adrenal function.

Pituitary ACTH-secreting tumors are treated with transphenoidal hypophysial microsurgery, irradiation, and, occasionally, medical suppressive therapy (with metyrapone, ketoconazole, aminoglutethimide, or mifepristone). Biologically active metastatic tumors are treated according to the patient's primary diagnosis.

Clinical Pearls

1. Cushing's syndrome is a constellation of signs and symptoms, not a disease. The differential diagnosis is lengthy, and a proper, comprehensive workup is required to ascertain the appropriate therapy.

2. All metabolically active, large, or potentially cancerous adrenal masses require surgical extirpation.

3. Biologically active adrenal tumors/adenomas tend to be ACTH-independent; in contrast, Cushing's disease and metastatic processes tend to be ACTH- or CRH-dependent.

REFERENCES

1. Novick AC, Howards SS: The Adrenals. In Gillenwater JY, Grayhack JT, Howards SS, Duckett JW (eds): Adult and Pediatric Urology, 3rd ed. St. Louis, Mosby-Year Book, Inc., 1996.
2. Daitch JA, Goldfarb DA, Novick AC: Cleveland Clinic experience with adrenal Cushing's syndrome. J Urol 158(6):2051–2055, 1997.
3. Vaughan ED: Diagnosis of surgical adrenal disorders. AUA Update Series 39(16):306–311, 1997.
4. Vaughan ED Jr, Blumenfeld JD: The adrenals. In Walsh PC, Retik AB, Vaughan ED, Wein AJ (eds): Campbell's Urology, 7th ed. Philadelphia, W.B. Saunders Company, 1998.

PATIENT 2

A 2-month-old child with a unilateral undescended testis

A 2-month-old child is referred to the urologist with a right-sided undescended testis. The diagnosis was made after normal vaginal delivery of a full-term 3.2-kilogram boy. The child has no siblings, but the father reports that he had an undescended testis as a child and had corrective surgery at the age of 3.

Physical Examination: General: well-nourished and active. Abdomen: soft, without masses. Genitalia: scrotum normal; phallus circumsized, with meatus in normal position; left testicle in scrotum, normal size and shape; right hemiscrotum empty, right testicle in inguinal canal; no dimples nor tufts of hair on sacrum (see figure).

Question: What is the most likely diagnosis, given the history and physical examination?

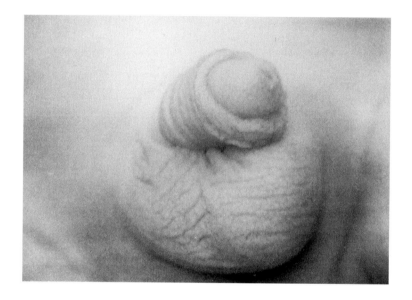

Diagnosis: Cryptorchidism

Discussion: Normal testicular descent results from an interaction between several hormonal and mechanical factors, including an intact hypothalamic-pituitary-testicular axis, intra-abdominal pressure, the genitofemoral nerve, and a normal gubernaculum. Some believe that cryptorchidism may be a mild form of hypogonadotropic hypogonadism.

The incidence of undescended testes in full-term boys is 3.4–5.8% and in premature boys 9.2–30%. At 3–6 months, 0.8–1.5% have an undescended testis, and descent beyond this point is rare. Undescended testes are more common in boys with low birth weight, a positive family history, hypospadias, spina bifida, and midline defects. Approximately 15% are bilateral. Potential locations of the testicle are abdominal (8%), inguinal (72%), and prescrotal–gliding or ectopic (20%). Nonpalpable testicles account for approximately 20% of undescended testicles.

Ectopic testicles are those that descend through the external ring but their final location is outside the descent path. These testicles usually are found in the superficial inguinal pouch and, occasionally, in the perineum, femoral canal, or the contralateral scrotum. Retractile testicles are found in boys 1–10 years of age. In these boys the testicle has undergone normal descent, but during examination it retracts into the inguinal canal because of an overactive cremasteric reflex. These testes are not considered undescended. These children present later because the cremasteric reflex is weak in infancy.

The patient should be examined in the frog-legged position in a warm room. One of the examiner's hands should be placed over the ipsilateral inguinal region of the undescended testicle, and the other hand should be used to examine the scrotum. This prevents retraction of the testicle with manipulation of the scrotum. If the testicle is not palpated in the scrotum, the hand over the inguinal canal can be used to locate and milk the testicle toward the scrotum with a lateral to medial motion.

The likelihood of histologic abnormality correlates with the amount of time the testicle remains in an abnormal location, and changes can occur as early as 6 months of age. Changes include a reduced number of germ cells and Leydig cells, impaired germ cell maturation, and hyalinization of the seminiferous tubules. In adult men, fertility is 85% after unilateral orchiopexy and 50–60% after bilateral orchiopexy. Risk of malignancy is four to ten times that of a normal testicle. Approximately 10% of testicular tumors in patients with cryptorchidism occur in the contralateral testicle. Because of the increased mobility of the testicle in the inguinal canal, it may undergo torsion if uncorrected. Seventy percent of undescended testicles are associated with a **patent process vaginalis**, which can result in an ipsilateral inguinal hernia.

Surgical treatment of the undescended testicle is performed to maximize the chance for fertility. Orchiopexy does not alter the risk of malignancy, but the ability to perform a testicular exam is improved with the testicle in the scrotum. Treatment should be initiated between 6–12 months of age. Testicles undescended by month 12 are unlikely to ever descend. Treatment in these cases is principally surgical.

The standard inguinal orchiopexy is begun with an incision over the inguinal canal. This incision is carried through the subcutaneous tissue and Scarpa's fascia to the external oblique fascia. The external oblique fascia is then opened in the direction of its fibers. Careful attention must be paid at this point to avoid injury to the ilioinguinal nerve. The testicle is identified in the tunics, and the gubernaculum is divided. The cord is skeletonized, segregating the cremasteric fibers and the process vaginalis from the cord structures. A high ligation of the process vaginalis is performed to prevent future hernias. These maneuvers usually provide sufficient length to deliver the testicle into the scrotum. If more length is required, the Prentiss maneuver may be required, in which the spermatic cord is brought medial to the inguinal canal by incising the internal inguinal ring medially and dividing the inferior epigastric vessels. The internal ring and the transversalis fascia are then closed lateral to the cord. Attention is now directed to the ipsilateral scrotum, where a 1-centimeter transverse incision is made in the mid scrotum. Through this incision, a subcutaneous dartos pouch large enough to accommodate the testicle is bluntly created. An opening in this pouch is sharply produced to allow access into the true scrotum. The testicle is then delivered into the true scrotum, through the window and into the dartos pouch. The neck of the dartos pouch can be closed around the cord with an absorbable stitch. This procedure is a dependable and successful means of orchiopexy that does not involve sutures placed in the testicle. The success rate of this procedure is approximately 98%.

Hormonal treatment consists of human chorionic gonadotropin and luteinizing hormone-releasing factor agonists together or individually. These treatments have been popular in Europe, but randomized controlled trials have failed to show significant benefit.

Laparoscopy or inguinal/abdominal exploration is the first step in treatment of the nonpalpable testicle. If the testis is nonpalpable, it is intra-abdominal in 50–80% of patients. Typically the remainder are atrophic, most commonly in the scrotum. This finding is due to in-utero torsion. Radiographic evaluation, such as ultrasound, is not helpful in patients with nonpalpable testicles. Computed tomography and magnetic resonance imaging are relatively accurate, but they do not significantly alter treatment.

Upon abdominal exploration, if the vessels enter the inguinal ring, then inguinal exploration is required. If the testicle is suspected to be nonviable, it should be removed to eliminate risk of malignancy. Findings of blind-ending vessels require no further exploration.

Intra-abdominal testicles are more difficult to place in the scrotum. Several surgical options are available, including the Prentiss maneuver with standard orchiopexy, the one- or two-stage Fowler-Stephens orchiopexy, microvascular autotransplantation, or orchiectomy. These procedures are being performed laparoscopically in some centers. The Fowler-Stephens orchiopexy consists of dividing the spermatic vessels and, therefore, the blood supply to the testicle from the cremaster and the artery of the vas deferens. After testicular mobilization, placement in the scrotum should be performed as previously described. Patients should be evaluated 1 year postoperatively and at puberty. The child should be instructed how to perform a self-examination.

The present patient was re-examined at 6 months of age and again was found to have a right undescended testis. He underwent a right orchiopexy at 9 months of age. Postoperative examination 6 weeks later revealed the testis to be in the scrotum and similar in size to the left testis.

Clinical Pearls

1. After orchiopexy, 85% of patients with unilateral and 50–60% of patients with bilateral undescended testicles are fertile.

2. Risk of malignancy is increased four- to tenfold in children with undescended testicles, and orchiopexy does not alter this risk.

3. With nonpalpable testes, 20–50% are absent secondary to in-utero torsion. Contralateral hypertrophy often is present in these boys.

4. Hormonal treatment for the undescended testicle has been ineffective in achieving testicular descent.

REFERENCES

1. Hrebinko RJ, Bellinger MF: The limited role of imaging techniques in managing children with undescended testes. J Urol 150:458–460, 1993.
2. Rozanski T, Bloom D: The undescended testis. Urol Clin North Am 22:107–118, 1995.
3. Elder JS: Evaluation and management of boys with a nonpalpable testis. In Elder JS (ed): Pediatric Urology for the General Urologist. New York, Igaku-Shoin, 1996.
4. Faerber GJ, Bloom DA: Pediatric endourology. In Gillenwater JY, Grayhack JT, Howards SS, Duckett JW (eds): Adult and Pediatric Urology, 3rd ed. Philadelphia, Mosby, 1996.
5. Kogan S, Hadziselimovic F, Howards SS, Snyder HM, Huff D: Pediatric andrology. In Gillenwater JY, Grayhack JT, Howards SS, Duckett JW (eds): Adult and Pediatric Urology, 3rd ed. Philadelphia, Mosby, 1996.
6. Rajfer J: Congenital anomalies of the testis and scrotum. In Walsh PC, Retik AB, Vaughan ED, Wein AJ (eds): Campbell's Urology, 7th ed. Philadelphia, W.B. Saunders, 1998.
7. Rozanski T, Bloom DA, Colodny A: Surgery of the scrotum and testis in children. In Walsh PC, Retik AB, Vaughan ED, Wein AJ (eds): Campbells Urology, 7th ed. Philadelphia, W.B. Saunders, 1998.

PATIENT 3

A 5-year-old boy with acute scrotal pain

A 5-year-old child is brought to the emergency department suffering from left scrotal pain of 6-hour duration. The pain began the day prior to presentation and has progressively increased over the last 24 hours. The patient denies trauma to the scrotum and testicle. The mother of the child reports no similar incidents. The child denies dysuria and abdominal pain, but reports nausea without emesis. No radiographic studies have been performed

Physical Examination: General: healthy appearing; moderate amount of distress. Abdomen: soft, without masses. Genitalia: normally positioned urethral meatus; right hemiscrotum mildly ecchymotic; right testicle normal size and position; left testicle approximately one and a half times the size of the right, but oriented in proper anatomic location in scrotum; left testicle exquisitely tender to palpation at upper pole.

Laboratory Findings: Urinalysis: unremarkable. WBC 9800/µl, normal differential.

Question: What is the diagnosis and treatment given the history and physical examination?

Diagnosis: Torsion of the appendix testis

Discussion: The appendix testis is a remnant of the mullerian duct. Located on the upper pole of the testicle, it possesses the ability to twist and infarct. The clinical significance of torsion of this appendage is that it must be distinguished from **testicular torsion**. Delay in the diagnosis of testicular torsion can result in significant consequences: testicular infarction can occur within 12–24 hours of torsion, and irreversible changes can occur in 3–6 hours, leading to loss of the testicle.

Torsion of the appendix testis is the most common cause of scrotal pain in children ages 2–10. Testicular torsion is the most common cause of scrotal pain in adolescent boys ages 12–18 and occurs in two thirds of that group. It accounts for 25–35% of the acute scrotal pain seen in the pediatric population. Males 12–18 years old with acute scrotal pain have testicular torsion at least 50% of the time.

In addition to testicular torsion, the differential diagnosis of torsion of the appendix testis includes acute epididymitis or torsion of the appendix epididymis. Other diagnoses that should be entertained with the acute onset of pain and swelling of the hemiscrotum are incarcerated inguinal hernia, testicular tumor, hydrocele, trauma, and hematocele.

Onset of pain in torsion of the appendix testis usually is gradual over a period of a day. Onset of pain in testicular torsion typically is over a period of hours. As with testicular torsion, children may report abdominal pain as well as nausea. Emesis is more common in the child with testicular torsion. Dysuria is not associated with either condition, but may be associated with acute epididymitis. Boys with torsion of the appendix testis usually do not report previous episodes of hemiscrotal pain that have resolved. In contrast, one third of boys with testicular torsion report previous episodes of pain. Intermittent torsion and spontaneous detorsion may account for these painful episodes.

Physical examination usually reveals a swollen scrotum, possibly with erythema, and a reactive hydrocele in both conditions. The testicle with a torsive appendix testis also features a distinct, tender, indurated mass near the upper pole. The classic **blue dot sign** over the point of tenderness is pathognomonic, but found infrequently. This finding is due to visualization of the infarcted appendix. In the case of testicular torsion, physical examination usually reveals a high-riding testicle with an abnormal orientation of its superior-inferior axis.

Urinalysis is without significant findings in both conditions, as opposed to the pyuria and bacteriuria seen in those with acute epididymitis. If the clinician desires, color Doppler sonography or testicular flow scan may be used to aid in the diagnosis. These studies show increased flow in the case of torsion of the appendix testis and diminished or absent flow in testicular torsion. If only 180–360 degrees of torsion are present, color Doppler ultrasound and testicular flow scans may be normal.

If the clinician is certain about the diagnosis of torsion of the appendix testis, then conservative treatment with anti-inflammatory agents and scrotal support is warranted. If there is any question about the diagnosis, immediate scrotal exploration should be carried out to exclude testicular torsion. *The viability of the testicle indirectly relates to the amount of time that it is ischemic.* With an aggressive approach to diagnosis and exploration, testicular salvage is 70% in cases of testicular torsion. Manual detorsion may be attempted prior to taking the patient to the operating room. This is performed by rotating the testicle on its superior-inferior axis in the outward direction (as viewed from the feet). If detorsion is successful, the patient experiences relief of his pain. Detorsion does not obviate the need for surgical correction, and prompt testicular fixation should be performed. After the testicle is detorsed, surgical exploration and orchiopexy of the contralateral testicle is done. The testicle in question then should be reassessed for viability. If the testicle appears dark and nonviable, orchiectomy is performed.

Clinical Pearls

1. In boys 2–10 years old, torsion of the appendix testis is the most common cause of acute scrotal pain.

2. In boys 12–18 years old, torsion of the testicle is the most common cause of acute scrotal pain.

3. The likelihood of testicular damage from torsion depends on the degree and duration of the torsion.

4. If the testicle is torsed < 360 degrees, a color Doppler ultrasound or testicular flow scan can appear normal.

5. Torsion of the appendix testis can be treated conservatively if the clinician is confident in the diagnosis.

REFERENCES

1. Kogan S, Hadziselimovic F, Howards SS, Snyder HM, Huff D: Pediatric Andrology. In Gillenwater JY, Grayhack JT, Howards SS, Duckett JW (eds): Adult and Pediatric Urology, 3rd ed. Philadelphia, Mosby, 1996.
2. Wainstein MA, Elder JS: Acute and chronic scrotal swelling. In Kliegman RM, Nieder ML, Super DM (eds): Practical Strategies in Pediatric Diagnosis and Therapy. Philadelphia, W.B. Saunders, 1996.
3. Rajfer J: Congenital anomalies of the testis and scrotum. In Walsh PC, Retik AB, Vaughan ED, Wein AJ (eds): Campbell's Urology, 7th ed. Philadelphia, W.B. Saunders, 1998.
4. Rozanski T, Bloom DA, Colodny A: Surgery of the scrotum and testis in children. In Walsh PC, Retik AB, Vaughan ED, Wein AJ (eds): Campbell's Urology, 7th ed. Philadelphia, W.B. Saunders, 1998.

PATIENT 4

A 16-month-old boy with an abdominal mass

A 16-month-old boy is referred to the urologist by his pediatrician for the evaluation of an abdominal mass. The mother notes that while bathing the child 1 month ago she observed a swelling in his abdomen. She denies difficulty with feeding or weight loss.

Physical Examination: General: no acute distress. Abdomen: left upper quadrant mass extending across the midline, firm and nontender. Liver: enlarged on palpation. Skin: multiple, blueish, nontender nodules on torso and extremities.

Laboratory Findings: CBC: mild anemia. Serum chemistry: normal. Computed tomography (CT) of abdomen: 11-cm suprarenal mass displacing left kidney inferiorly and extending across midline; three large nodules in liver appear metastatic.

Question: What is the likely diagnosis given the presentation and laboratory findings?

Diagnosis: Neuroblastoma

Discussion: Neuroblastoma is the most common tumor of infancy, accounting for approximately 6–8% of childhood malignancies. Fifty percent of the tumors occur in children less than 2 years old, and 75% occur in children less than 4 years old. There is a 2% incidence of associated brain and skull defects, yet other abnormalities are not associated with the neuroblastoma. Twenty percent of the tumors arise in children with an inheritable mutation.

The neuroblastoma cells arise from the same cells that form the sympathetic ganglia and adrenal medulla: the neural crest cells. Other tumors from the same cell line that are related to neuroblastoma are the ganglioneuroma and ganglioneuroblastoma.

The tumor is surrounded by a pseudocapsule, and when cut it appears gray. It is lobulated and may contain cystic components. Histologically, the cells may be arranged in pseudorosettes. The cells show characteristics reflective of their neural tube origin, including dendritic appendages and granules containing catecholamines. The tumor can arise anywhere along the sympathetic chain, most commonly in the abdomen, but also in the head, neck, chest, and pelvis. Paravertebral tumors may extend into the spine. Celiac or abdominal masses tend to do the most poorly. Adrenal and retroperitoneal masses do as well as those arising in other sites.

Patient survival is inversely correlated with age at diagnosis. Younger children also have a higher rate of spontaneous regression. Other factors that relate poorly to prognosis include higher tumor stage, N-myc expression, elevated ferritin levels, DNA ploidy, and the amount of stroma contained in the tumor.

The presentation depends on the location of the tumor. The majority of the tumors arise in the abdomen (> 50%); two thirds of these occur in the adrenal gland. Patients typically present with a large, irregular abdominal mass that extends across the midline. Pain usually is not a factor. The differential diagnosis includes other abdominal and retroperitoneal tumors. Metastasis is found in 70% of patients at the time of presentation, typically in the liver or bone. Children with neuroblastoma present with a poorer clinical picture than those with Wilms' tumor because of the likelihood of early metastasis. Symptoms include malaise, fever, weight loss, difficulty feeding, and anemia. In infants, the tumor preferentially disseminates to the liver; in older children, bone is the preferential site of metastasis. The long bones and skull are common sites. Bone marrow is involved in 50% of patients. **Subcutaneous blue nodules** also are not uncommon, occurring in one third of infants with the disease. Children may have periorbital metastases that give the appearance of proptosis and ecchymosis. Symptoms rarely are attributed to the release of catecholamines by the tumor. Vasoactive intestinal peptide can be released, causing diarrhea. Children with metastatic disease may have anemia secondary to bone marrow replacement. Bone marrow biopsy is indicated in all patients with neuroblastoma.

Two major catecholamine metabolites are found in 90% of the 24-hour urine collections of patients with neuroblastoma: **homovanillic acid** and **vanillymandelic acid**. Despite the high levels of these metabolites, these patients typically do not present with hypertension or elevated levels of norepinephrine. The norepinephrine is broken down in the tumor, unlike pheochromocytoma, in which the catecholamine is released into the blood.

Chest x-ray and abdominal CT should be performed to determine the extent of the disease. The chest radiograph should be examined for extension through the diaphragm and to rule out lymph node, rib, and vertebral metastases. A skeletal survey is indicated because of the high incidence of bony metastasis. These lesions often are lytic. Nuclear bone imaging studies also may be indicated. Plain films of the abdomen show the characteristic **stippled calcifications** of the tumor 50% of the time. Magnetic resonance imaging can be used to evaluate the involvement of the major vessels and the spine.

Neuroblastoma Staging

Stage 0	Neuroblastoma in situ
Stage I	Tumors confined to the organ or structure of origin
Stage II	Tumors extending in continuity beyond the organ or structure of origin but not crossing the midline; the regional lymph nodes on the ipsilateral side may be involved
Stage III	Tumors extending in continuity beyond the midline; regional lymph nodes may be involved bilaterally
Stage IV	Distant metastases involving bones, bone marrow, brain, skin, liver, lung, soft tissues, or distant lymph node groups
Stage IV-S	Patients who would otherwise be classified with stage I or II disease but who have remote spread of tumor confined to one or more of the following sites: liver, skin, or bone marrow (without radiographic evidence of bony metastases on complete skeletal survey)

Tumors undergo spontaneous regression in 1–2% of patients with neuroblastoma. The disease falls into two distinct groups (see table). Patients with favorable disease are those with stage I, II, or IV-S disease. Their overall disease-free survival is 89% at 2 years. Those with unfavorable disease, stage III or IV, require an aggressive, multimodal treatment regimen. Surgical removal of disease is the treatment of choice in children with stages I and II disease. Surgery also is useful in staging the disease. Debulking of tumors has minimal effect on treatment outcome. Neither chemotherapy nor radiotherapy is needed in the group of patients with favorable disease. However, surgery may be delayed until after chemotherapy has rendered the tumor operable in those with unfavorable disease. Neuroblastoma is a chemoresponsive tumor, and chemotherapy alone or with bone marrow transplant is a mainstay in the treatment of patients with stage III or IV disease. Radiation also is an important part of many of the treatment regimens for these patients, and it can be used for palliation, as well.

Finally, patients with stage IV-S disease (8–12% of children with the disease) make up a special group of patients. These children are observed for some time before any therapy is instituted because of the high rate of regression of these tumors. Chemotherapy and radiation therapy may be used to palliate symptoms while waiting for regression.

Clinical Pearls

1. Neuroblastoma is the most common tumor of infancy, accounting for approximately 6–8% of childhood malignancies.

2. The neuroblastoma cells arise from the same cells that form the sympathetic ganglia and adrenal medulla.

3. Homovanillic acid and vanillymandelic acid are found in the urine in 90% of the 24-hour urine collections of patients with neuroblastoma.

REFERENCES

1. Ritchey ML, Andrassy RJ, Kelalis PP: Pediatric urologic oncology. In Gillenwater JY, Grayhack JT, Howards SS, Duckett JW (eds): Adult and Pediatric Urology, 3rd ed. Philadelphia, Mosby, 1996.
2. Snyder HM, D'Angio GJ, Evans AE, Raney RB: Pediatric oncology. In Walsh PC, Retik AB, Vaughan ED, Wein AJ (eds): Campbell's Urology, 7th ed. Philadelphia, W.B. Saunders, 1998.

PATIENT 5

A newborn girl with an abdominal mass

A one-hour-old, full-term, female infant is presented for a urology consultation to evaluate a palpable right abdominal mass. No prenatal care was obtained.

Physical Examination: Vitals: normotensive. Abdomen: soft, nondistended; right mass not crossing the midline and not fixed; mass transilluminates. Genitalia: normal.

Laboratory Findings: Abdominal radiograph: displacement of small bowel to left. Ultrasound: severe right-sided hydronephrosis with no obvious ureteral dilation, thin-appearing renal parenchyma, left kidney normal (see figure).

Questions: What is the differential diagnosis of an abdominal mass in a newborn? What further workup is needed in this child?

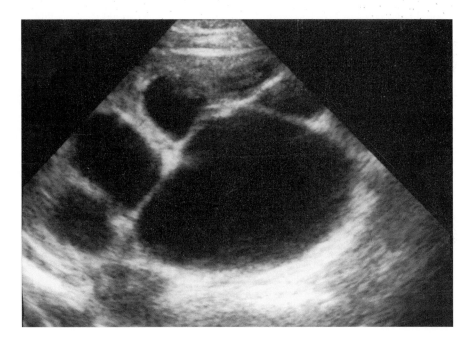

Diagnosis: Ureteropelvic junction obstruction

Discussion: A palpable abdominal mass in a newborn is considered a **urologic emergency** requiring expeditious evaluation. Of such findings, 50–70% are urologic in origin and require surgical intervention.

The differential diagnosis of a neonatal abdominal mass is extensive, but initially can be broken down into masses that are fluid-filled (or cystic) and those that are solid. The more common lesions are cystic, with ureteropelvic junction obstruction and multicystic kidneys accounting for 35–45% of all neonatal masses. The most common solid lesions include neuroblastoma, mesoblastic nephroma, and, rarely, Wilms tumor.

Important elements of the history include prenatal documentation of oligohydramnios or intrauterine hydronephrosis. Many neonatal lesions are identified antenatally by ultrasound. This child was unfortunate, in that no prenatal care was obtained.

The initial physical examination of any neonate should include a thorough abdominal assessment. When a mass is appreciated, particular note should be made of its location, laterality, mobility, and transillumination properties. A lower abdominal mass suggests a distended bladder secondary to posterior urethral valves in a male, or hydrometrocolpos in a female. A mass that crosses the midline and feels fixed suggests neuroblastoma. Bilateral flank masses could be secondary to distal obstruction, bilateral ureteropelvic junction obstruction, or autosomal recessive polycystic kidney disease.

The radiologic evaluation of a neonatal abdominal mass should start with an ultrasound of the abdomen. A plain film also is important to evaluate possible intestinal obstruction, obvious soft tissue lesions, or calcifications. A neuroblastoma can appear as a paravertebral soft tissue mass, with classic punctate calcifications. Ultrasound alone can provide an accurate diagnosis in most cases.

The present patient had obvious unilateral hydronephrosis and healthy, though thin-appearing, ipsilateral renal parenchyma. Although a ureteropelvic junction obstruction was suggested by ultrasound, a voiding cystourethrogram was done to rule out the possibility of reflux, and a MAG-3 diuretic renal scan was performed to assess parenchymal function and collecting system washout. (An argument could be made for a dimercaptosuccinic acid technetium-99 [DMSA-Tc99] instead of the MAG-3.) The voiding cystourethrogram showed no evidence of reflux. The MAG-3 diuretic renal scan showed a differential function of 25% on the involved side, with an obstructed pattern on the washout portion of the study ($t\frac{1}{2} > 60$ min).

A **dismembered pyeloplasty** was performed at 2 months of age. Pathologic examination of the specimen revealed the obstructing segment to be composed of disorganized, circular, smooth muscle, with an increased ratio of collagen to smooth muscle fibers. A follow-up renal scan at 8 months showed no evidence of obstruction, with nearly equal differential renal function.

Clinical Pearls

1. A palpable abdominal mass in a newborn should be considered a surgical emergency, and a urologic consultation should be obtained promptly.

2. Ureteropelvic junction obstruction is the most common cause, followed by a multicystic dysplastic kidney. Solid lesions are less common, and include neuroblastoma, mesoblastic nephroma, and, rarely, Wilms tumor.

3. The initial radiologic exam should include plain abdominal films and an abdominal ultrasound. Ultrasound can provide an accurate diagnosis in most cases.

4. A voiding cystourethrogram should be obtained when a hydronephrotic kidney is seen on ultrasound, to rule out vesicoureteral reflux. A functional study (MAG-3 renal scan) also should be performed.

5. Dismembered pyeloplasty is the treatment of choice for ureteropelvic junction obstruction in neonates and infants, and has a high success rate.

REFERENCES

1. Hanna MK, Jeffs RD, Sturgess JM, Barkin M: Congenital UPJ obstruction and primary obstructive megaureter. J Urol 116:725–730, 1976.
2. Snyder HM III, Lebowitz RL, Colodny AH, et al: UPJ obstruction in children. Urol Clin North Am 7:273–290, 1980.
3. Wilson DA: Ultrasound screening for abdominal masses in the neonatal period. Am J Dis Child 136:147–151, 1982.
4. Diamond DA: Hydrometrocolpos. Society for Pediatric Urology Newsletter, March 1988.
5. Hartman GE, et al: Abdominal mass lesions in the newborn: Diagnosis and treatment. Clin Perinatol 16(1):123–125, 1989.
6. Elder JS: Antenatal hydronephrosis: Fetal and neonatal management. Pediatr Clin North Am 44(5):1299–1321, 1997.

PATIENT 6

A 12-year-old boy with flank pain and fever

A 12-year-old boy is brought to his pediatrician with a 2-day history of fever and left flank pain. Upon further questioning the child admits to some dysuria and urgency, but denies any incontinence. He goes on to describe three similar episodes with left-sided pain and fever in the past.

Physical Examination: Temperature 39°. Abdomen: soft, no distension, no masses; mild fullness at left flank with costovertebral angle tenderness. Genitalia: normal; no urethral discharge, no epididymal tenderness. Rectal: normal tone; no evidence of impaction.

Laboratory Findings: Urinalysis: > 10 WBC/hpf, 5–10 RBC/hpf, many bacteria. Urine cultures: pending. Ultrasound: severe hydroureteronephrosis on left.

Questions: What is your diagnosis? What further workup is needed?

Diagnosis: Recurrent pyelonephritis with left-sided megaureter

Discussion: The megaureter, or wide ureter, is a radiographic finding, not a single defined pathologic entity. The finding of a wide ureter in a young child requires further radiologic investigation for functional characterization. The common classification of the wide ureter includes three types: (1) refluxing megaureter, (2) obstructed megaureter, and (3) nonrefluxing-nonobstructed megaureter. Two important studies to clarify this delineation are the **voiding cystourethrogram** to assess a refluxing component and the **diuretic renal scan** to assess an obstructing component.

The obstructed megaureter, or what is sometimes referred to as the primary-obstructed megaureter, is three to four times more common in boys and three to four times more common on the left. The etiology of this lesion is not clear. Microscopically, there is an increase in the ratio of collagen to smooth muscle, and this smooth muscle often is disorganized. Grossly, the distal ureter is not found to be stenotic, as evidenced by the easy passage of a ureteral catheter past the involved segment. These microscopic and gross findings have led some to hypothesize that the functional obstruction is the result of a failure of the distal ureter to dynamically propagate ureteral peristalsis (i.e., adynamic segment theory).

It is interesting to note that 10% of contralateral kidneys can be either absent or dysplastic in the presence of an obstructed megaureter. This underscores the importance of the renal scan in the workup of a megaureter.

The present patient underwent a voiding cystourethrogram, which was found to be normal, i.e., no refluxing component. He then underwent a diuretic MAG-3 scan which showed 30% relative function on the left, with a T1/2 prolonged beyond 30 minutes during the diuretic portion of the study. This result was consistent with an obstructed-type megaureter. Left-sided ureteral tapering with reimplantation was performed, as described by Hendren in 1969. At 1-year followup, no further urinary tract infections were documented by culture, and a renal scan showed no evidence of obstruction.

Clinical Pearls

1. A megaureter is a radiographic description, and it requires further investigation to classify it functionally.

2. The wide ureter can be classified into a refluxing type, an obstructed type, and a non-refluxing-nonobstructed type.

3. The primary obstructed megaureter is three to four times more common in boys and three to four times more common on the left.

4. The etiology of the obstructed megaureter is uncertain; however, the theory of an adynamic segment is certainly a plausible one.

5. The treatment of choice for the obstructed megaureter is an antirefluxing ureteroneocystostomy, with ureteral tapering as indicated for redundant tissue.

REFERENCES
1. Hendren WH: Operative repair of megaureter in children. J Urol 101:491, 1969.
2. Tanagho EA, Smith DR, Guthrie TH: Pathophysiology of functional ureteral obstruction. J Urol 104:73, 1970.
3. Baskin LS, Zderic SA, Snyder HM, Duckett JW: Primary dilated megaureter: Long-term follow-up. J Urol 152:618–621, 1994.

PATIENT 7

A 6-year-old girl with fever, flank pain, and incontinence

A 6-year-old girl is brought to her pediatrician with a 1-day history of fever and right flank pain. Her mother says she has wet the bed the last two nights and was incontinent of urine at school yesterday. On questioning, the child admits to some burning on urination and denies any previous episodes.

Physical Examination: Temperature 38.6°. Abdomen: soft, no masses, no distension. Extremities: moderate right flank tenderness. Genitalia: normal, no discharge. Rectal: normal tone, no evidence of impaction.

Laboratory Findings: Urinalysis: elevated leukocyte esterase, elevated nitrite, many bacteria.

Question: What is your diagnosis?

Diagnosis: Pyelonephritis, first episode

Discussion: The incidence of urinary tract infection during the first year of life is greater in boys. During this time, roughly 2.5% of boys experience urinary tract infection, compared to 0.7% of girls. Most affected boys are uncircumcised. By school age, the numbers are dramatically different: less than 1% of boys have a urinary tract infection, compared to 1–3% of girls. Interestingly, 4–7% of all visits to the pediatrician for fever uncover urinary tract infection as the cause.

Urinary tract infections in children can be classified into three groups: pyelonephritis, cystitis, and asymptomatic bacteriuria. These infections are ascending, with the offending bacteria from the child's feces. Pyelonephritis (kidney infection) is characterized by fever, abdominal or flank pain, and occasionally nausea/vomiting. Cystitis (bladder infection) is characterized by dysuria, urgency, frequency, incontinence, suprapubic pain, and/or malodorous urine. Asymptomatic bacteriuria is rare.

The diagnosis of a urinary tract infection in an older child can be straightforward if irritative symptoms (e.g., dysuria, urgency, frequency) predominate. However, voiding dysfunction in the form of diurnal enuresis may be the only presentation. Occasionally these children have a history of constipation; therefore, they should be questioned about their bowel habits. The infant and toddler usually present with fever and irritability.

The urinalysis is key in making the presumptive diagnosis of a urinary tract infection. There are four specimen types: bagged, voided, catheterized, and aspirated. The diagnostic yield of a bagged specimen is poor, and a catheterized or suprapubically aspirated specimen should be obtained from any child that is not toilet trained in whom a urinary tract infection is suspected. Urine culture is necessary for diagnosis. However, if both the leukocyte esterase and nitrite are positive, the sensitivity of urinalysis is nearly 100%. Conversely, the negative predictive value of urinalysis is 95% if both are negative.

The strategy in management of pediatric urinary tract infections is to treat the acute episode with appropriate antibiotics and mimimize the risk of renal injury. This is accomplished by identifying those children with an anatomic/functional predisposition to urinary tract infections and either treating them definitively or providing appropriate prophylaxis. In a septic child with pyelonephritis, initial intravenous administration of a broad-spectrum agent(s) for urinary pathogens should be administered (ampicillin plus gentamicin, cefazolin plus gentamicin, or ceftriaxone) for 2–4 days, followed by a 10- to 14-day course of an appropriate oral agent (cephalexin, trimethoprim-sulfamethoxazole (TMP), amoxicillin). The patient should be maintained on antibiotic prophylaxis until radiologic evaluation is complete.

As mentioned, prophylaxis is warranted in the child awaiting evaluation. Other indications include: normal urinary anatomy with frequent urinary tract infections (two or three per year), vesicocoureteral reflux, urethral instrumentation, and clean intermittent catheterization. The ideal prophylactic drug is well tolerated, with low serum levels, high urinary levels, and minimal effect on fecal flora. Nitrofurantoin and TMP-SMX often are used. Nitrofurantoin should not be used in children with glucose-6-phosphodiesterase deficiency, as it can precipitate a hemolytic anemia, and TMP-SMX should not be used in the first 2 months of life because it can exacerbate the physiologic hyperbilirubinemia of neonates.

The indications for radiologic evaluation in children are: all those less than 5 years old, all boys (regardless of age), all girls with a febrile urinary tract infection (regardless of age), and girls older than 5 with a second urinary tract infection. Renal ultrasound and a voiding cystourethrogram are routinely ordered. If an abnormality is identified, a dimercaptosuccinic acid–technetium-99 (DMSA-Tc99) renal scan may help assess the impact of the lesion on renal function.

In the present patient, oral antibiotic therapy was initiated, with adjustment following culture and sensitivity results. She was found to have grade III/V vesicoureteral reflux of the right system, with no other abnormalities. She was placed on TMP-SMX prophylaxis, with plans to repeat a culture every 4 months for 18 months and obtain a radionuclide cystogram and ultrasound in 18 months to reassess her reflux.

Clinical Pearls

1. Young children presenting with irritative voiding symptoms should be questioned about incontinence and bowel habits. They may present with only diurnal enuresis, or have a history of constipation.

2. A catheterized or aspirated specimen should be obtained from a child who is not toilet trained in whom a urinary tract infection must be ruled out. A bagged specimen may yield a false positive result.

3. In children, it is of primary importance to identify any anatomic/functional predisposition to urinary tract infection, so that pyelonephritic scarring (reflux nephropathy) can be prevented.

4. Antibacterial prophylaxis is indicated in the child awaiting radiologic evaluation; with normal anatomy and frequent urinary tract infections; with vesicoureteral reflux; who has undergone urethral instrumentation; and who receives intermittent catheterization.

5. Radiologic evaluation is indicated in the child who is less than 5 years old, all boys (regardless of age), all girls with a febrile urinary tract infection (regardless of age), and all girls older than 5 with a second urinary tract infection.

REFERENCES

1. Stamey TA: A clinical classification of urinary tract infections based upon origin. South Med J 68:934, 1975.
2. Hardy J, Furnell P, Brumfitt W: Comparison of sterile bag, clean catch, and suprapubic aspiration in the diagnosis of urinary infection in early childhood. Br J Urol 48:279–283, 1976.
3. Lohr J, Portilla M, Geuder T, et al: Making a presumptive diagnosis of UTI by using a urinalysis performed in an on-site lab. J Pediatr 122:22–25, 1993.
4. Clarke SE, et al: Technetium-99m-DMSA studies in pediatric urinary infection. J Nucl Med 37(5):823–828, 1996.
5. Rushton HG: Urinary tract infections in children: Epidemiology, evaluation, and management. Pediatr Clin North Am 44(5):1133–1169, 1997.

PATIENT 8

A 40-year-old man with bloody urethral discharge

A 40-year-old man presents with a 2-week history of a bloody, purulent urethral discharge. He complains of dysuria, urinary urgency, and frequency of urination. He has nocturia four times each evening. He has no complaints of decreased force of stream, incontinence, or prior urinary tract infections. He has no history of recent instrumentation to the urinary tract or prior surgical history. This is his first episode with this complaint, and he is quite anxious. He is not married and has had unprotected sexual intercourse with four women over the last 6 months.

Physical Examination: Pulse 72; blood pressure 130/70. Cardiac, chest, abdomen: normal. Genitalia: circumcised; purulent discharge from urethral meatus; penis otherwise normal and nontender; testicles normal size and consistency, with left spermatocele. Rectum: normal; no suspicion of prostate infection or neoplasm.

Laboratory Findings: Gram-stain of urethral swab: gram-negative cocci. Cultures on Thayer-Martin media: *Neisseria gonorrhoeae*. *Chlamydia trachomatis* detected by polymerase chain reaction. Urine culture: no growth.

Question: What recommendations would you give this patient for treatment and prevention?

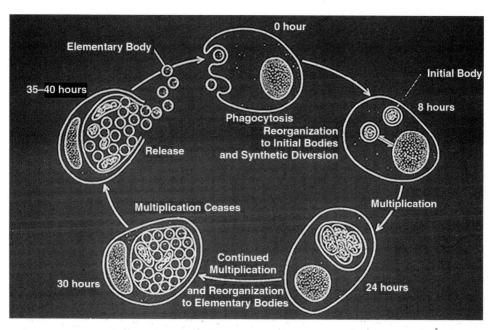

Life cycle of *Chlamydia trachomatis*.

Diagnosis: Urethritis secondary to both *Neisseria gonorrhoeae* and *Chlamydia trachomatis*

Discussion: It is important to recognize that urethritis can be caused by more than one organism simultaneously. For a man, the risk of acquiring gonococcal urethritis after one episode of unprotected sex with a women infected with the bacteria is 17%. With increased unprotected sexual experiences, the risk of this transmission increases greatly. Gonococcal urethritis can be present and asymptomatic in 40–60% of partners of patients with gonorrhea. The diagnosis of gonorrhea is made with a urethral swab—a drop of urethral discharge should *not* be used. Gram-negative cocci are identified on a Gram stain, and confirmed on culture using Thayer-Martin media.

Chlamydia trachomatis can be recovered from the urethra in 4–35% of men with gonococcal urethritis. *C. trachomatis* is an intracellular parasite of columnar epithelium. Its usual incubation period is 1–5 weeks following intercourse. Asymptomatic infection is common.

The treatment of gonococcal urethritis is one dose of intramuscular ceftriaxone (250 milligrams). Alternative regimens include one dose of spectinomycin 2 grams intramuscularly or ciprofloxacin 500 milligrams. Penicillin should be avoided because many penicillinase-producing organisms have evolved. The treatment of urethritis secondary to *C. trachomatis* includes 7 days of tetracycline 500 milligrams four times daily, doxycycline 100 milligrams twice daily, or erythromycin 500 milligrams four times daily. It is also important to screen all sexual partners of the patient for the presence of these organisms and provide appropriate treatment.

This patient received both ceftriaxone and doxycycline. His symptoms subsided, and he has not suffered any recurrent episodes or sequelae to date. He was advised to use condoms when having sexual intercourse to decrease the risk of acquiring another sexually transmitted disease.

Clinical Pearls

1. *Neisseria gonorrhoeae* and *Chlamydia trachomatis* can coexist and cause urethritis (4–35% of men).
2. Despite the presence of both organisms, the patient may be asymptomatic.
3. All partners of the contact patient should be screened and treated appropriately.
4. Protected intercourse must be stressed.

REFERENCES

1. Keck C, Gerber-Schafer C, Clad A, et al: Seminal tract infections: Impact on male fertility and treatment options. Hum Reprod Update 4(6):891–903, 1998.
2. van Duynhoven YT, Schop WA, van der Meijden WI, van de Laar MJ: Patient referral outcome in gonorrhoea and chlamydial infections. Sex Transm Infect 74(5):323–330, 1998.
3. Duncan B, Hart G: Sexuality and health:The hidden costs of screening for *Chlamydia trachomatis*. BMJ 318(7188):931–933, 1999.
4. Palladino S, Pearman JW, Kay ID, et al: Diagnosis of *Chlamydia trachomatis* and *Neisseria gonorrhoeae*: Genitourinary infections in males by the Amplicor PCR assay of urine. Diagn Microbiol Infect Dis 33(3):141–146, 1999.

PATIENT 9

A 57-year-old man with recurrent urinary tract infections and pneumaturia

A 57-year-old man presents with a 6-week history of urinary frequency and urgency, with the passage of small bubbles, especially at the termination of urination. His urine has become odiferous and he has passed small amounts of mucous over the past week.

Physical Examination: Vital signs: normal. Abdomen: soft, with active bowel sounds; mild left lower quadrant tenderness to deep palpation, but no rebound tenderness nor peritoneal signs; no masses; bladder not full to percussion. Genitalia: normal. Prostate: smooth, soft, nontender.

Laboratory Findings: WBC 12,000/μl, normal differential. Serum creatinine 1.4 mg/dl. Urinalysis: many leukocytes, few red blood cells, positive nitrite, trace protein. Barium enema: see figure.

Question: What is your diagnosis?

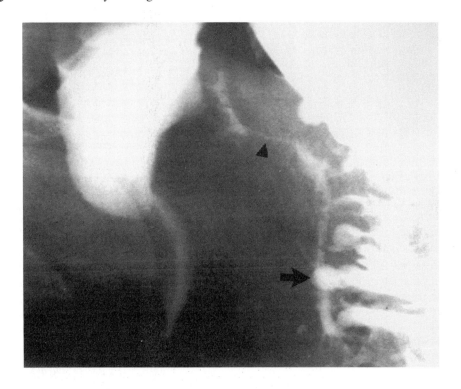

Diagnosis: Colovesical fistula

Discussion: A colovesical fistula is a communication that has developed between the enterics and the bladder. The communication can develop because of persistent irritation, inflammation, iatrogenic injury, foreign body, or malignancy. The symptom of pneumaturia is considered pathognomic for this condition. However, only 43–63% of patients exhibit this symptom; many do not demonstrate pneumaturia, despite the presence of a fistula. Another finding consistent with this diagnosis is fecaluria, but it, too, is not always present. In men, the only alternative ways of introducing air into the bladder are via gas-forming organisms or iatrogenic means, such as irrigation of a foley catheter. In women, sexual activity also can introduce air.

The patient's age is pertinent to this scenario. The age range of 45 to 70 is common for pathology to strike the bowel or bladder. Diseases to consider include microperforations of the bowel, diverticulitis of the sigmoid colon, bladder cancer, and colon cancer. Urinary tract infections are considered abnormal in a man in this age range; if discovered, they should be pursued aggressively. If the infections are recurrent and of various organisms, a communication with the bowel should be considered, even in the absence of pneumaturia. Of patients with a colovesical fistula, 75% have a history of urinary tract infection. Many patients complain only of irritable bladder symptoms.

The evaluation of the patient with a colovesical fistula is somewhat controversial. No study is 100% accurate in making the diagnosis. Studies that are of limited usefulness are: ingestion of activated charcoal to check the urine for its presence, cystoscopy (77% accurate), cystogram with voiding phase (34%), barium enema (34%), and computed tomography (CT) with contrast of the abdomen and pelvis. All of these studies may fail to show the fistula. However, the CT scan is most useful for demonstrating bowel pathology or regions of inflammation near the wall of the bladder. An intravenous pyelogram usually is not helpful.

Repair of a colovesical fistula usually is a combined effort between general surgery and urology. Prior to operating, both the gastrointestinal and the genitourinary tracts must be sterilized. Exploration is performed via a midline incision, affording the best exposure. General surgery performs the bowel resection at the region of pathology, and the required reanastomosis or colostomy. Urology repairs the bladder. The fistula tract should be excised completely, leaving a 1- to 2-centimeter margin of normal tissue on the specimen. Intraoperative ureteral stents may be useful to identify the ureter to avoid injury. The bladder is excised back to healthy tissue, then closed in a standard two-layer fashion with absorbable suture. Interposition of omentum between bowel and bladder repair, placement of a closed suction drain at the operative site, and placement of a large-caliber Foley catheter complete the procedure. The catheter may be removed in 5–7 days.

In the present patient, a fistula and sigmoid diverticulitis were demonstrated on CT scan. This evidence coupled with the symptom of pneumaturia pinpointed the diagnosis. Surgery, as described above, was performed with success.

Clinical Pearls

1. Pneumaturia most often indicates a colovesical fistula.

2. Multiple modalities may be required to make the diagnosis.

3. The preoperative preparation requires sterilized gastrointestinal and genitourinary tracts.

4. Operative therapy, with careful attention to possible malignancy, is the treatment of choice.

REFERENCES

1. Shatila A, Ackerman N: Diagnosis and management of colovesical fistulas. Surg Gynecol Obstet 143:71, 1976.
2. Carson C, Malek R, Remire W: Urologic aspects of vesicoenteric fistulas. J Urol 119:744, 1978.
3. Goldman S, Fishman E, Gatewood C, Seigelman S: Computed tomography in the diagnosis of enterovesical fistulae. Am J Radiol 144:1229, 1985.
4. Freiha F: Surgical treatment of enterovesical fistulas. In Walsh PC, Retik AB, Stamey TA, Vaughan ED Jr (eds): Campbell's Urology, 6th ed. (Vol. 3). Philadelphia, W.B. Saunders Co., 1992, pp 2771–2774.

PATIENT 10

A 22-year-old woman with dysuria, frequent urination, and hematuria

A 22-year-old woman presents with a 2-day history of urinary urgency, frequency, and hematuria. She reports pain on initiation of urination. She had a similar problem approximately 6 months ago that cleared with antibiotics. She denies flank pain or fever. She denies any prior urologic surgery or history of difficulties as a child.

Physical Examination:　Vital signs: normal. Abdomen: soft, with mild suprapubic tenderness; no masses palpable. Extremities: no flank tenderness. Pelvic exam: slightly erythematous urethral meatus.

Laboratory Findings:　WBC 6700/μl, normal differential. Urinalysis: leukocytes, red blood cells too numerous to count, nitrite negative, pH 6.0, moderate protein. Urine culture: no bacterial growth; urinary sediment contains epithelial cells with intranuclear inclusion bodies.

Question:　What is your diagnosis?

Diagnosis: Acute cystitis

Discussion: Acute cystitis is inflammation and infection of the lower urinary tract, which can be caused by a variety of offending agents including bacteria, viruses, yeast, chemicals, allergic reactions, and instrumentation. The triad of symptoms described in young women may be associated with acute viral cystitis. Viral lesions tend to be more hemorrhagic than bacterial lesions, and they usually are self-limited. Viral cystitis typically is caused by adenoviruses type 11 and 21 or papovirus.

Symptoms usually resolve in 2–3 weeks, even without treatment. The etiology of viral cystitis is controversial, but is presumed to be hematogenous spread. A full urologic evaluation is unnecessary if the diagnosis of viral cystitis is made. The diagnosis can be confirmed via urinary sediment analysis, with intranuclear inclusion bodies within epithelial cells.

The differential diagnosis should include urethral syndrome or bacterial cystitis. Urethral syndrome is characterized by frequency and dysuria without bacteriuria. Of patients with urethral syndrome, 40% can be documented to have positive cultures of the upper tracts. Radiographic evaluation generally is not indicated, unless the patient is a child. Bacterial cystitis usually is documented by a positive urine culture with an identifiable organism. The bacteria are from the Enterobacteriaceae family (87% *Escherichia coli*), but also 4% *Staphylococcus saprophyticus*, 3% *Proteus mirabilis*, and 3% Klebsiella. *E. coli* of the O antigen serotype and those containing type I fimbriae promote attachment of bacteria to the bladder wall, by adhering to bladder mucin or trapping via uromucoid.

Both urethral syndrome and acute bacterial cystitis are conventionally treated with a 7–10 day course of antibiotics. Quinolones should not be considered first-line.

In the present patient, the diagnosis was confirmed by the presence of intranuclear inclusion bodies in her epithelial cells. Successful resolution of her cystitis occurred within 7 days.

Clinical Pearls

1. Viral cystitis is hemorrhagic more often than nonviral cystitis.
2. Inclusion bodies in the urine sediment are used to make the diagnosis of viral cystitis.
3. Spread likely occurs via hematogenous transfer.
4. Urethral syndrome and bacterial cystitis should be considered in the diagnosis.
5. O antigen and type I fimbriae promote bladder wall attachment.

REFERENCES

1. Busch R, Huland H: Correlation of symptoms and results of direct localization in patients with urinary tract infections. J Urol 132:282, 1984.
2. Freedman L: Natural history of urinary infection in adults. Kidney Int 96(suppl 4), 1974.
3. Stamey T: Pathogenesis and Treatment of Urinary Tract Infections. Baltimore, Williams and Wilkins, 1980.
4. Schaeffer A: Infections of the urinary tract. In Walsh PC, Retik AB, Stamey TA, Vaughan ED Jr (eds): Campbell's Urology, 6th ed. (Vol. 3). Philadelphia, W.B. Saunders, 1992, pp 731–806.

PATIENT 11

A 59-year-old man with urinary tract infection and swelling, ulceration, and necrosis of scrotal skin

A 59-year-old man with a past medical history significant for diabetes mellitus presents to the emergency department with dysuria and acute onset of scrotal swelling. He recently underwent a circumcision due to recurrent paraphimosis. His family states that he has been acting oddly for the past 2 days; for example, calling his wife of 30 years by a different name.

Physical Examination: Temperature 38.9°; pulse 110; respirations 29; blood pressure 109/68. Genitalia: foreskin incision erythematous, with some wound separation; scrotum erythematous, swollen, and malodorous, with pain and crepitus on palpation.

Laboratory Findings: WBC 16,000/μl, with left shift on differential. Urine dipstick: nitrite positive, leukocyte esterase positive, glucose positive. Microscopic urinalysis: significant bacteriuria and WBC. Blood and urine cultures: pending.

Questions: What is the likely diagnosis? What management would you recommend?

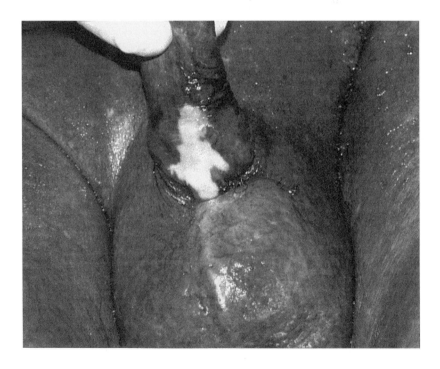

Answer: Fournier's gangrene, requiring immediate and aggressive surgical debridement and triple antibiotics

Discussion: Fournier's gangrene is a form of necrotizing fasciitis that presents as a progressive, fulminating infection about the male genitalia. First described by Baurienne in 1764 and Fournier in 1883, this infection most commonly arises in skin in the urethral or rectal regions. Predisposing factors include diabetes mellitus, local trauma, steroid use, immunosuppression, paraphimosis, periurethral extravasation of urine, and surgeries, including circumcision. When originating in the genitalia, the infection spreads along Buck's fascia of the penis, dartos fascia of the penis and scrotum, Colles' fascia of the perineum, and Scarpa's fascia of the anterior abdominal wall.

On physical exam, early presentation may be limited to induration of the penis or scrotal skin. However, with progression, erythema and crepitus may extend over the perineum and abdominal wall. Dysuria, urethral discharge, and obstructive voiding symptoms may exist. A fetid, feculent odor may be present, suggestive of anaerobic infection. Sepsis can occur, resulting in alterations in mental status, tachypnea, and tachycardia. The clinical differentiation between necrotizing fasciitis and cellulitis may be difficult at early presentation. However, systemic toxicity out of proportion to local findings points to Fournier's gangrene as the more likely diagnosis.

Fournier's gangrene is a urologic emergency requiring immediate, wide surgical debridement of the involved skin and subcutaneous tissue, as well as areas beyond. A diverting colostomy may be required if a colonic source is suspected. Urinary diversion by suprapubic catheter may be necessary with urethral stricture or urinary extravasation. The wound should be packed open, with a second procedure/excision in 24–48 hours if necrosis or infection continues. Antibiotic coverage should be broad-based, including ampicillin, gentamicin, and metronidazole.

Mortality ranges from 20–50%, with higher mortalities in diabetics, alcoholics, and those with colorectal sources of infection. These latter patients tend to present later, with more extensive disease.

The present patient underwent emergent, wide surgical debridement and was started on triple antibiotics. He died of gram-negative sepsis on postoperative day 2.

Clinical Pearls

1. Fournier's gangrene is a urologic emergency requiring immediate surgical attention.
2. Predisposing factors include: diabetes mellitus, immunosuppression, periurethral/anal infections, local trauma, and paraphimosis.
3. Mortality ranges from 20–50%.

REFERENCES
1. Spirnak JP, Resnick MI, Hampel N, Persky L: Fournier's gangrene: Report of 20 patients. J Urol 131:289–291, 1984.
2. Paty R, Smith AD: Gangrene and Fournier's gangrene. Urol Clin North Am 1:149, 1992.
3. Schaffer AJ: Infection in the urinary tract. In Walsh PC, Retik AB, Vaughan AD Jr, Wein AJ (eds): Campbell's Urology, 7th ed. Philadelphia, W.B. Saunders, 1998, pp 533–605.

PATIENT 12

A 52-year-old man with inflammation of the foreskin

A 52-year-old man with a recent history of uncontrolled noninsulin-dependent diabetes mellitus presents with a 3-day history of circumferential inflammation of the distal foreskin. The inflammation extends slightly into the inner prepuce. The patient claims the inflammation is aggravated and burns with urination. Also, the lesion minimally bleeds with aggressive retraction of the foreskin. He denies ever having a similar lesion in the past.

Physical Examination: Genitalia: long prepuce, with an erythematous, distal, "rash-like" lesion (see figure); lesion associated with mild edema, tender to palpation, and extends slightly into inner prepuce; glans, shaft, and remainder of genital skin normal. Lymph nodes: no inguinal lymphadenopathy.

Laboratory Findings: Complete blood count: normal. Blood glucose: 440 mg/dl. Urinalysis: excess protein and glucose.

Questions: What is your diagnosis? Which disorders are part of the differential?

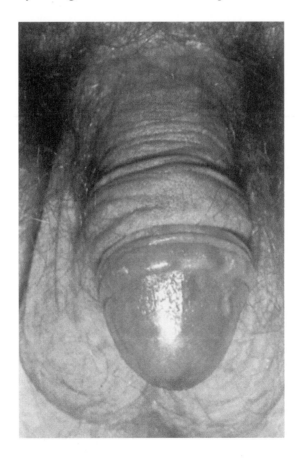

Diagnosis: Candidal fungal infection of the foreskin. Other major diagnostic considerations include balanitis xerotica obliterans, leukoplakia, erythroplasia of Queyrat, and dermatitis.

Discussion: This patient's presentation is typical of fungal infection of the foreskin, especially with the history of diabetes mellitus. Occasionally, this fungal infection is the presenting sign of diabetes mellitus due to the large amount of glucose spilling into the urine. Glucosuria and a long prepuce causes fungal, mainly *Candida albicans*, overgrowth involving the prepuce or glans (i.e., balanitis), secondary to trapping of urine after urination.

Candida is an opportunistic pathogen in the presence of predisposing risk factors, which include diabetes mellitus, malignancy, obstructive uropathy, neurogenic dysfunction, and congenital anomalies. Furthermore, antibiotic therapy, steroids, and immunosuppressive therapy enhance a patient's vulnerability. Candidal infection most commonly involves the prepuce or glans, but the distal urethra, rarely, also may be involved. Initially, it may present as an erythematous rash that itches and burns upon urination. Fissures may be present in the reddened area. It may progress to superficial erosions, pustules, and white patches on the glans or prepuce. However, in the vulnerable patient, superficial infections can become invasive. For instance, emphysematous cellulitis of the penis has been caused by *C. albicans* in a diabetic patient without early treatment. All of these lesions may be pruritic.

Diagnosis depends on physical, microscopic, and potassium hydroxide (KOH) examinations. Microscopic examination of the lesion/exudate reveals inflammatory cells among which can be identified budding yeast forms and pseudohyphae. After the KOH has had adequate time to digest keratin, the mycelia and spores of Candida should be apparent. Culture can be helpful, but seldom is required for diagnosis.

Treatment consists of controlling the metabolic dysfunction, such as hyperglycemia, and discontinuing the broad-spectrum antibiotics in an effort to resolve the localized candidal colonization. Appropriate topical antifungal therapy, such as fluconazole or miconazole, also is important. In addition, retraction of the foreskin while urinating may help with hygienic control of the fungal overgrowth.

If conservative treatment and topical antifungal agents do not resolve the infection in an appropriate time period, a biopsy may be needed to rule out more serious and invasive diseases of the penis. Furthermore, repeated fungal infection predisposes the patient to phimosis, which places the patient at risk for additional infections. In order to break this vicious cycle, a circumcision may be necessary to prevent spread of infection and to reduce the risk of more invasive infections or cancer.

In the present patient, KOH examination revealed *C. albicans*. Control of his diabetes and 30 days of topical therapy with fluconazole successfully eliminated his fungal infection.

Clinical Pearls

1. Candidal penile infections can be easily treated with topical antifungals.
2. The primary etiologic cause must be resolved to prevent repeat infections.
3. A prophylactic circumcision may be needed.

REFERENCES
1. Wise GJ: Genitourinary candidal infection. American Urology Association Update Series 8(25):194, 1989.
2. Lynch DF, Schellhammer PF: Tumors of the penis. In Walsh PC, Retik AB, Vaughan ED, Wein AJ (eds): Campbell's Urology, 7th ed. Philadelphia, W.B. Saunders, 1998, p 2453–2485.

PATIENT 13

A 45-year-old man with an ulcerated lesion on his foreskin

A 45-year-old man presents with a 5-day history of a lesion on his foreskin. The lesion initially began as a reddish papule, which subsequently eroded. It is painless and slightly "oozy." The patient has a history of unprotected sex in the past month with a partner with known sexually transmitted diseases.

Physical Examination: Genitalia: solitary, painless ulceration on foreskin; borders smooth and sharply defined; entire lesion indurated; lesion size less than 0.5 centimeters. Inguinal lymph nodes: enlarged, hard, and nonsuppurating.

Laboratory Findings: Complete blood count, electrolytes, and urinalysis: normal. Rapid plasma reagin (RPR) test: reactive. Venereal Disease Research Laboratory (VDRL) test: negative. Darkfield examination: see figure.

Question: What is the differential diagnosis?

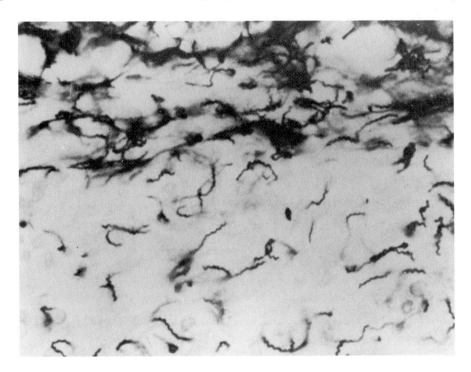

Diagnosis: Primary syphilis; diagnostic considerations include genital herpes, carcinoma-in-situ (e.g., erythroplasia of Queyrat, Bowen's disease) with malignant transformation or penile carcinoma

Discussion: Syphilis is an acute and chronic infectious disease caused by *Treponema pallidum.* It usually is acquired by sex and sex play during the infectious period. The disease passes through a primary stage, which is manifested by a chancre (an ulceration at the point of inoculation); a secondary stage, with systemic symptoms, adenopathy, and rash; an early latent stage, which is an asymptomatic period of variable duration with reactive serologic tests; and, finally, a late stage involving the the mucocutaneous, osseous, visceral, cardiovascular, and neural systems.

The primary stage appears after an incubation period of approximately 3 weeks. It is characterized by a chancre that emerges at the point of inoculation. The chancre begins as a papule and soon erodes and becomes ulcerative. It characteristically is painless, indolent, punched-out, and clean, with a scanty, yellow, serous discharge. The borders of the ulcer are raised, smooth, and sharply defined; the base is finely granular and hard; and the entire lesion is indurated. The neighboring lymph nodes are discretely enlarged, hard, and nonsuppurating. Most chancre of the penis occurs on the prepuce, coronal sulcus, glans, or frenulum.

The diagnosis of primary syphilis is established by discovery of *T. pallidum* on darkfield examination and by the reagin and treponemal blood tests. The RPR test usually is reactive by day 7 of the chancre. The VDRL test may not be positive in this time period and may need to be repeated. In 2–6 weeks, the chancre heals without treatment, and the patient progresses to the secondary stage.

The drug of choice for the treatment of syphilis is penicillin, usually benzathine penicillin G 2.4 million units intramuscularly, weekly for two doses. Those who are allergic to penicillin are given doxycycline 100 milligrams orally every 12 hours for 14 days. Following treatment, all patients with primary syphilis should be nonreactive at 12 months.

Other causes of infectious genital ulcer disease include genital herpes, which is the most common sexually transmitted genital ulcer disease in North America, followed by primary syphilis. The manifestations of genital herpes are highly variable; however, this disease typically is described as a group of vesicles that quickly ulcerate, resulting in multiple, shallow, *painful* ulcers. Acyclovir is the drug of choice for treatment. Topical, intravenous, and oral forms are effective for genital herpes.

Premalignant lesions such as Bowen's disease and erythroplasia of Queyrat also can eventually cause ulcerations on the penis. Both of these variants of carcinoma in situ feature a red, sometimes velvety, well-marginated lesion on the glans or foreskin. Diagnosis is made by biopsy. Microscopically, these lesions are similar, but erythroplasia of Queyrat is not associated with the high incidence of systemic neoplasia that is found in patients with Bowen's disease. There also is a 92% detection rate of the human papillomavirus (HPV), mainly HPV-16 and HPV-18, in carcinoma in situ. Treatment includes circumcision and topical 5-fluorouracil. Failures of topical chemotherapy can be salvaged with Mohs surgery or laser therapy.

In the present patient, repetition of the VDRL test produced a positive result, and darkfield examination revealed *T. pallidum.* He was treated with benzathine penicillin G and 12 months later was nonreactive. Additionally, he was counseled on protection against sexually transmitted diseases.

Clinical Pearls

1. Infectious genital ulcer disease most commonly involves herpes or syphilis lesions.
2. Ulcers refractory to conservative treatment must be biopsied to rule out carcinoma in situ or penile carcinoma.

REFERENCES
1. Cupp MR, Malek RS, Goellner JR, Smith TF, Espy MJ: The detection of human papillomavirus deoxyribonucleic acid in intraepithelial, in situ, verrucous and invasive carcinoma of the penis. J Urol 54:1024–1029, 1995.
2. Fiumara NJ: The diagnosis and treatment of infectious syphilis. Compr Ther 21(11):639–644, 1995.
3. DiCarlo RP, Martin DH: The clinical diagnosis of genital ulcer disease in men. Clin Infect Dis 25:292–298, 1997.

PATIENT 14

A 61-year-old man with an ulcer on his glans penis

A 61-year-old man presents with an 8-month history of an ulcerative lesion of the glans penis. The initial lesion, which was a small excrescence with a rough surface, was diagnosed as a wart. No treatment was performed. The lesion became eroded and, after 2–3 months, clearly ulcerated. The ulcer slowly increased in size, but was painless. Six months after the initial lesion, he noted small, marble-like lesions in the inguinal region.

Physical Examination: Genitalia: grossly oval-shaped, 2-centimeter ulcerative lesion on glans penis; lesion has granular, bleeding surface, with an infiltrated base and hard edges. Inguinal lymph nodes: lymphadenopathy and numerous small, firm, mobile nodules noted bilaterally.

Laboratory Findings: Red and white blood cell counts: normal. Biochemical work-up, urinalysis, chest radiograph: normal. Venereal Disease Research Laboratory (VDRL) test: negative.

Question: What disorder is indicated by the characteristics of these lesions?

Diagnosis: Squamous cell carcinoma of the penis

Discussion: In the United States and Europe, penile cancer is a rare neoplasm, accounting for 0.4–0.6% of all male malignancies. It may constitute 10–20% of all male cancers in some African and South American countries.

Squamous cell carcinoma accounts for about 95% of all penile malignancies. It usually presents in the sixth decade of life, and its incidence is directly related to cultural procedures such as circumcision that avoid the chronic irritative effects of smegma. These effects predispose a patient to penile carcinoma. Exposure to smegma is accentuated by phimosis, which is found in 25–75% of patients with penile cancer.

The first symptom of penile cancer usually is the appearance of a painless, exophytic growth—an ulcerated nodule or a flat ulcer that does not heal, but enlarges progressively. It can develop in any anatomic location of the penis, such as the glans (48%), prepuce (21%), both glans and prepuce (9%), coronal sulcus (6%), and shaft (less than 2%).

A penile lesion that does not respond to a short trial of conservative treatment requires a biopsy to confirm the diagnosis of penile carcinoma. In addition, the penile lesion is assessed with regard to size, location, fixation, and involvement of the corporeal bodies, and rectal and bimanual examinations are performed to rule out invasion or the presence of a pelvic mass. Careful bilateral palpation of the inguinal area is of extreme importance since the strongest prognostic indicator for survival is the presence or absence of nodal metastasis. However, 50% of palpable nodes are found to contain cancer, and 15% of clinically normal nodes contain unsuspected metastasis. Hence, a patient with palpable inguinal nodes should be re-examined 4–6 weeks after antibiotic therapy, to enhance staging accuracy, *before* imaging studies or lymphadenectomy is contemplated.

The most commonly used penile cancer staging classification is Jackson's classification: stage I, tumor limited to the glans and/or prepuce; stage II, tumor invading the shaft of the penis; stage III, tumor with operable inguinal metastasis; stage IV, tumor invading adjacent structures, or with inoperable nodes of distant metastasis.

The laboratory examination in patients with penile cancer typically is normal. Computed tomography and magnetic resonance imaging of the abdomen/pelvis or ultrasonography of the penis and/or inguinal nodes may be of some help in detecting pelvic node invasion, inguinal node metastasis, or local extent of the penile lesion.

The gold standard of therapy for penile cancer is partial or total penectomy. For lesions involving the glans and distal shaft, even when superficial, a partial amputation with resection 2 centimeters from the proximal margin of the tumor is necessary to minimize recurrence. If an adequate 2-centimeter margin cannot be achieved, or the lesion invades the corpora, or the phallic stump prevents normal voiding, a total penectomy is mandatory, followed by perineal urethrostomy. Circumcision is sufficient treatment for carcinoma in situ and small stage I cancers entirely limited to the foreskin. The disfigurement that occurs with penile amputation has popularized efforts toward organsparing techniques, such as partial excision or Moh's micrographic surgery, as well as nonsurgical therapies for smaller noninvasive lesions, such as radiation, laser (CO_2, YAG), or cryodestruction.

Since carcinoma of the penis is among the few malignancies for which removal of both the primary and draining lymphatics is of therapeutic value, radical ilioinguinal lymphadenectomy remains the mainstay for treating locally metastatic penile cancer. Unfortunately, the morbidity associated with this extensive dissection (i.e., phlebitis, pulmonary embolus, wound infection, flap necrosis, and disabling lower extremity and scrotal edema) makes the selection of patients that would benefit from this procedure of paramount importance. It is helpful to refer to an algorithm for managing inguinal nodes following the diagnosis of squamous cell carcinoma (see figure).

In the present patient, due to the extensive changes in the initial lesion over an 8-month period, a biopsy was performed immediately. It confirmed the diagnosis, and antibiotic therapy was begun to assist in staging. After 4 weeks, re-examination led to a determination of stage I cancer, and a partial penectomy was performed.

Algorithm for Management of Inguinal Nodes in Squamous Carcinoma of Penis

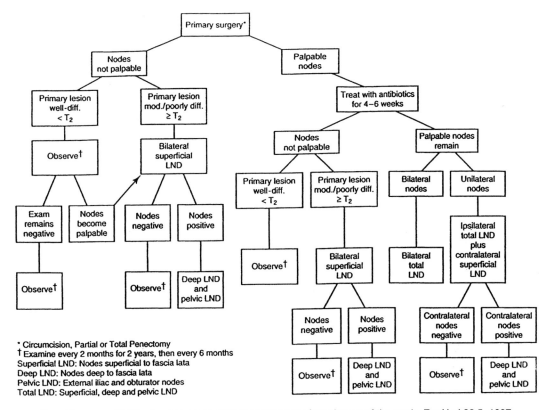

From Pizzocaro G, Piva L, et al: Up-to-date management of carcinoma of the penis. Eur Urol 32:5, 1997.

Clinical Pearls

1. A high index of suspicion for penile carcinoma and a low threshold for biopsy of all penile lesions that do not respond to a short trial of conservative therapy are of prime importance for early diagnosis and treatment of patients with carcinoma of the penis.

2. Survival is related to stage.

3. Ilioinguinal lymphadenectomy can be of therapeutic value.

REFERENCES

1. Burgers JK, Badalament RA, Drago JR: Penile cancer: Clinical presentation, diagnosis, and staging. Urol Clinics North Am 19(2):247, 1992.
2. Pizzocaro G, Piva L, et al: Up-to-date management of carcinoma of the penis. Eur Urol 32:5, 1997.
3. Schubach A, Cuzzi-Maya T, et al: An ulcerative lesion of the penis. Arch Dermatol 133:1303, 1997.
4. Lynch DF, Schellhammer PF: Tumors of the penis. In Walsh PC, Retik AB, Vaughan ED, Wein AJ (eds): Campbell's Urology, 7th ed. Philadelphia, W.B. Saunders, 1998, p 2453–2485.

PATIENT 15

An 83-year-old man with a scrotal mass

An 83-year-old man presents to his primary care physician with a complaint of an enlarged left testicle. The patient states that the testicle had progressively enlarged over the past month, but he was not concerned because it was not painful. The patient denies any voiding symptoms, trauma, and prior genitourinary pathology. The patient also reports a recent weight loss of 10 pounds and states that he has been sleeping about 12 hours per day. Past medical history is significant for mild hypertension.

Physical Examination: Genitalia: scrotum enlarged without any superficial edema or erythema; left testis grossly enlarged; right testis normal to palpation; right testicle 2-centimeter diameter, left testicle 6-centimeter, both normal shape and contour with no masses palpable; epididymis and spermatic cords normal. Genitourinary system: otherwise normal.

Laboratory Findings: HCT 41%, WBC 12,000/μl with normal differential, platelets 233,000/μl. Hemoglobin 13.7 g/dl. Alpha fetoprotein (AFP), beta-human chorionic gonadotropin (b-HCG), lactic acid dehydrogenase levels: normal. Urinalysis: normal. Ultrasound of scrotum: diffusely enlarged left testis, normal-size right testis; parenchyma homogenous throughout, with no masses; no increase in blood flow in testes (see figure). Chest radiograph and computed tomography (CT) scan of abdomen: normal.

Question: What is the most likely diagnosis?

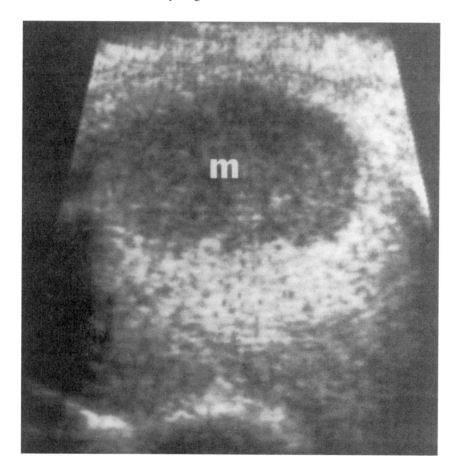

Diagnosis: Lymphoma

Discussion: The first steps in assessing a patient with enlarged testes are an adequate history and a thorough physical examination. The results should key the clinician in on the diagnosis. Epididymitis may cause testicular swelling, but it usually is accompanied by pain and an abnormal urinalysis. Scrotal masses always should create suspicion for malignancy. Ultrasound is the most frequently used diagnostic modality, along with the serum tumor markers AFP and b-HCG. Peak incidences for testicular tumors occur in late adolescence to early adulthood (20–40 years), in late adulthood (over 60 years), and in childhood (0–10 years).

Germ cell tumors of concern include seminoma, embryonal carcinoma, teratoma, choriocarcinoma, and yolk sac tumors. Non-germ cell tumors include Leydig-cell tumors, Sertoli-cell tumors, gonadoblastoma, adenocarcinoma of the rete testis, and carcinoid and mesenchymal tumors. Secondary tumors include leukemia, lymphoma, and metastasis from solid tumors at other sites (i.e., adenocarcinomas of the prostate, lung, kidney, and gastrointestinal tract, and melanoma). Secondary tumors are known to occur predominantly in men over 50 years old; lymphoma is the most common of these malignancies. In general, seminoma is rare after age 60. Spermatocytic seminoma, representing 10% of all seminomas, presents most often after age 50.

Lymphoma constitutes approximately 5% of all testicular tumors, with a median age of occurrence of approximately 60 years. It is the most frequent of all testis tumors in patients older than 50. The testis is painless and diffusely enlarged, with a diameter of 4 to 5 centimeters or more. Histologic study reveals a bulging, gray or pink lesion with ill-defined margins. There often is hemorrhage and necrosis present. Diffuse histiocytic lymphoma is the most common microscopic finding, although all varieties have been identified. Those patients with lymphocytic types tend to survive longer than those with histocytic types. Generalized constitutional symptoms, including weight loss, weakness, and anorexia, occur in 25% of patients. Bilateral tumors occur in about 50% of patients, with 10% occurring simultaneously. Most patients present with occult disseminated disease, and for this reason the cornerstone of treatment is systemic chemotherapy. Treatment of primary testicular lymphoma should include radical orchiectomy.

Lymphoma of the testis can be seen as a late manifestation of widespread lymphoma, an initial presentation of clinically occult disease, or primary extranodal disease. Survival is poor with bilateral disease and poor in patients with lymphoma at other sites who later experience a testicular relapse. Investigation should include a complete blood count, peripheral smears, bone marrow studies, chest x-ray, and bone scan. Intravenous pyelogram, CT scan, lymphogram, and liver and spleen scans are useful in staging. Retroperitoneal staging is essential in the assessment, and decisions to do retroperitoneal lymphadenopathy are dependent on the individual clinical situation, the institution, and discussions with the medical oncologist.

In the present patient, the left testicle was enlarged with no masses identified, as is typical of lymphoma. He underwent a radical orchiectomy for primary testicular disease. Histologic examination revealed a bulging, gray lesion of uncertain borders consistent with diffuse histiocytic lymphoma. He was begun on a course of systemic chemotherapy, with no evidence of recurrence on a 3-month followup visit.

Clinical Pearls

1. Scrotal masses always should create suspicion of malignancy.
2. Painless enlargement of a testicle in an elderly male always should lead to the suspicion of lymphoma.
3. Retroperitoneal staging is essential in the workup of lymphoma.
4. Lymphoma is the most common secondary neoplasm of the testis and the most frequent of all testis tumors in patients over 50 years of age.

REFERENCES
1. Connors JM, Klimo P, Voss N, et al: Testicular lymphoma: Improved outcome with early brief chemotherapy. J Clin Oncol 6:776–781, 1988.
2. Walsh PC, Retik AP, Stamey TA, Vaughan ED (eds): Campbell's Urology, 7th ed. Philadelphia, W.B. Saunders, 1998.

PATIENT 16

A 61-year-old man with gross hematuria

A 61-year-old man presents to his doctor with a chief complaint of "blood in my urine." The patient denies any medical problems, works as an accountant, and generally considers himself healthy. He states that he has never been hospitalized. The patient denies alcohol or drug use, but admits to smoking "half a pack" of cigarettes per day since age 16. He denies voiding difficulty and claims to have good flow of urine.

Physical Examination:　General: relatively healthy. Abdomen: no tenderness. Genitourinary system: normal.

Laboratory Findings:　Urinalysis: pink urine with more than 100 red blood cells per high-power field; otherwise unremarkable. Urine culture: negative for infection. Urine cytology: positive for atypical cells. Intravenous pyelogram: normal upper tracts; irregular filling defect along left lateral wall of bladder (see figure).

Question:　What is the most probable diagnosis?

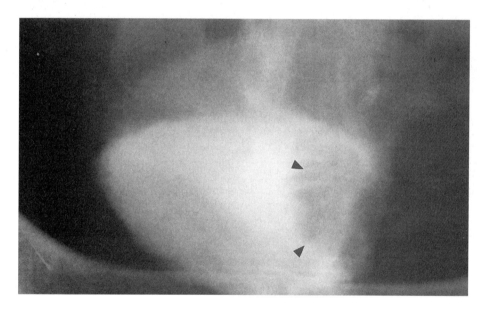

Diagnosis: Transitional cell carcinoma of the bladder

Discussion: Gross painless hematuria in a male always should elicit concern for bladder cancer. Other causes of hematuria include infection, stones, benign prostatic hyperplasia, renal parenchymal lesions, renal pelvis tumors, trauma, and benign idiopathic hematuria. Urinary cytology is helpful in diagnosing carcinoma in situ and other high-grade lesions. Some urologists use DNA cytometry or newer urine-based assays instead of cytology. Patients with hematuria always should undergo radiologic imaging. Intravenous pyelography is the gold-standard imaging study in evaluating hematuria. Other options include ultrasound or CT scan, in select circumstances. Direct cystoscopic examination is required to rule out bladder pathology.

Bladder cancer is a frequently encountered diagnosis in urology. The incidence of bladder cancer is on the rise, and more than 90% of new cases are transitional cell carcinomas. Male-to-female ratio is 3:1. The average ages are 69 years for males and 71 years for females, and the incidence of bladder cancer increases directly with age. Etiologic factors associated with bladder cancer include cigarette smoking, metabolites of aniline dyes, aromatic amines, nitrosamines, tryptophan metabolites, pelvic irradiation, cyclophosphamide, arsenic, chlorinated water, and shistosomiasis (squamous cell carcinoma). Workers in the chemical, dye, rubber, petroleum, leather, and printing industries are at increased risk; however, cigarette smoking remains the strongest risk factor, accounting for up to 50% of cases.

Transitional cell carcinomas most commonly appear as papillary exophytic lesions and, less commonly, sessile and ulcerated lesions. Transitional cell carcinoma has a great metaplastic potential, with up to one third containing spindle cell, squamous cell, or adenocarcinoma elements. A strong correlation exists between tumor grade and stage. Grading is rated from 0 to 3 based on cell size, pleomorphism, nuclear polarization, hyperchromatism, and the number of mitoses present. Stage and grade are inversely proportional to prognosis.

Staging System for Transitional Cell Carcinoma

Stage	Finding
Ta	Papillary tumor invading only mucosa
Tis	Carcinoma in situ
T1	Invasion of lamina propria
T2	Superficial muscle infiltration
T3a	Deep muscle infiltration, but confined to muscularis
T3b	Invasion through muscle into perivesical fat
T4	Invasion into adjacent organs

Treatment of transitional cell carcinoma is dependent on the stage of the tumor. Superficial tumors are effectively treated with transurethral resection and surveillance. Patients with unresectable superficial tumors, carcinoma in situ, or several recurrences should be considered for additional therapy. The most commonly used therapy is intravesical bacille Calmette-Guérin. Other intravesical therapies include mitomycin C, thiotepa, etoglucid, and doxorubicin. Alternatively, some centers use oral therapy with bropiramine or megadose vitamins, TP40, or intravesical interferon. Newer modalities being studied include intravesical keyhold limpet hemocyanin, intravesical gene therapy, and photodynamic therapy. Cystectomy for superficial disease is considered only if there is diffuse, unresectable tumor or carcinoma in situ that does not respond to intravesical chemotherapy.

Recommended follow-up includes cystoscopy and cytology every 3 months for 24 months, then every 6 months for an additional 2 years, then annually thereafter. Positive cytology is considered a recurrence, and an aggressive search for recurrent tumor should be made in the entire urinary tract. Radiologic surveillance should be routinely performed; however, the most beneficial frequency is unclear. A yearly intravenous pyelogram is considered by many to be adequate for radiologic surveillance.

Muscle-invasive bladder tumors are initially treated with transurethral resection. Tumors with limited muscle invasion may be cured with this treatment; however, in most cases muscle-invasive tumors should be treated with cystectomy and urinary diversion. Transitional cell carcinoma involving the prostatic urethra and high-grade tumors of the bladder neck require a concomitant urethrectomy. Partial cystectomy may be considered for solitary invasive tumors in a location such as the dome of the bladder, where adequate margins can be achieved. Chemotherapy has been used with limited success both as neoadjuvant or adjuvant chemotherapy. Metastatic disease usually is treated with platinum-based chemotherapy. The most commonly used regimen is MVAC (methotrexate, vinblastin, doxorubicin, and cisplatin). Radiation also is used, on a palliative basis and occasionally as definitive therapy with salvage cystectomy.

In the present patient the intravenous urogram demonstrated marked irregularity of the left lateral wall, consistent with invasive disease. This was confirmed on cytoscopy, CT scan, and subsequent bladder biopsy. The patient was found to have T3a disease and was treated with a radical cystoprostatectomy and neobladder. Followup at 1 year revealed normal upper tracts and no evidence of recurrence.

Clinical Pearls

1. Gross painless hematuria in an elderly male always should elicit concern for bladder cancer.

2. Intravenous pyelography is the gold-standard imaging study in evaluating hematuria.

3. Stage and grade of transitional cell carcinoma are inversely proportional to prognosis.

4. Superficial transitional cell carcinoma is effectively treated with transurethral resection and surveillance.

5. Muscle-invasive transitional cell carcinoma often requires cystectomy and urinary diversion.

REFERENCES

1. Tanagho EA, McAninch JW (eds): Smith's General Urology, 14th ed. Norwalk, Appleton and Lange, 1996.
2. King WD, Marrett LD: Case-control study of bladder cancer and chlorination by-products in treated water (Ontario, Canada). Cancer Causes Control 7(6):596–604, 1996.
3. Ismail MT, Lattime EC, Gomella LG: Current management of superficial bladder cancer: BCG and beyond. Monographs Urol 19(3):33–55, 1998.
4. Walsh PC, Retik AP, Stamey TA, Vaughan ED (eds): Campbell's Urology, 7th ed. Philadelphia, W.B. Saunders, 1998.

PATIENT 17

A 53-year-old man with microscopic hematuria

A 53-year-old man is found to have microscopic hematuria on routine physical examination. The patient is otherwise healthy. He has a 35-year history of smoking approximately 1–2 packs of cigarettes per day. He drinks 1–2 cups of coffee per day. There is no history of occupational exposure to carcinogenic agents. He reports no excessive intake of phenacitin or other, related agents.

Physical Examination: Unremarkable.

Laboratory Findings: Intravenous urogram: 2-centimeter, round filling defect in right renal pelvis, with incomplete filling of upper pole infundibulum and calyces (see figure). Urinalysis: RBC 10/hpf. Cytology: neoplastic and atypical cells.

Question: What is the differential diagnosis for a kidney filling defect on intravenous urogram?

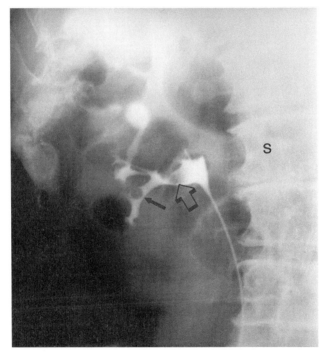

Air bubble (*thin arrow*) and filling defect (*wide arrow*).

Answer: A filling defect in the kidney can be caused by a stone, tumor, blood clot, fungus ball, sloughed papilla, or vascular impression.

Discussion: Renal pelvis tumors account for approximately 10% of all renal tumors and about 5% of all urothelial tumors. Approximately 30–75% of patients with upper tract urothelial tumors have bladder tumors at some time. Transitional cell carcinoma accounts for more than 90% of upper tract urothelial tumors. Other tumors occurring in the upper tract include squamous cell carcinoma, adenocarcinoma, inverted papilloma, sarcoma, neurofibromas, small cell carcinoma, angiosarcomas, and fibroepithelial polyps.

Many risk factors have been identified. The strongest risk comes from smoking, with a threefold increase. Individuals who drink more than 7 cups of coffee per day have a risk of 1.8 for developing transitional cell carcinoma. Phenacitin use and abuse has been well documented as a risk factor. In fact, phenacitin abuse and coexisting papillary necrosis can increase the risk by 20-fold. Cyclophosphamide and its metabolite, acrolein, have been identified as risk factors. Also identified are occupational exposures to chemicals, petro chemicals, and plastics, as well as coal, coke, asphalt, and tar. Chronic infections, irritation, and calculi may slightly increase risk. Upper tract transitional cell carcinoma has been associated with the Lynch syndrome II and Balkan nephropathy.

Diagnosis usually is achieved through a combination of intravenous urography, urinary cytology, and endoscopic confirmation. In 10–30% of patients, the tumor causes obstruction or nonvisualization of the collecting system on intravenous urogram. Computed tomography (CT) scan without intravenous contrast may be useful in distinguishing solid masses from uric acid stones, which are radiolucent on standard urography. Cystoscopy is necessary to rule out any bladder tumors. Bilateral involvement in 2–5% of cases requires contralateral evaluation. If the bladder appears normal, then retrograde pyelograms and selective cytology can confirm the diagnosis. If the diagnosis is not conclusive, ureteroscopy may be performed. Approach to the tumor may be percutaneous or retrograde, with a biopsy or resection of the lesion.

Tumor stage can be used to predict prognosis, with a median survival of 97 months for low-stage tumors and 13 months for high-stage tumors. CT scan often is helpful in determining local spread or the presence of metastasis. However, CT scan often fails to detect multifocal lesions. Spread is thought to occur via epithelial, lymphatic, and hematogenous dissemination.

Upper tract transitional cell carcinoma tends to recur unilaterally; thus, the gold-standard treatment is nephroureterectomy with resection of a bladder cuff. Laparoscopic nephroureterectomy has been advocated as a feasible treatment option. Some investigators recommend resecting low-grade tumors through ureteroscopic or antegrade approaches. Adjuvant therapy with bacille Calmette-Guérin, mitimycin-C, and thiotepa has been used to prevent recurrences with uncertain efficacy. Cystoscopy is a mainstay of followup due to the downward seeding that occurs with upper tract transitional cell carcinoma.

Radiation therapy has been used with some benefit, mainly for high-grade or invasive lesions. Chemotherapeutic regimens are the same as those used in bladder cancer. MVAC therapy (methotrexate, vinblastin, doxorubicin, cisplatin) has been disappointing, with a complete response rate of 5–10%. Angioinfarction also may be used in certain situations when a symptomatic lesion presents in patients with diffuse metastasis or when patients are not candidates for immediate nephrectomy because of comorbidity.

In the present patient, ureteroscopy confirmed the presence of a papillary transitional cell carcinoma of the right renal pelvis. No other uretal abnormalities were noted. He underwent a nephroureterectomy, and pathologic examination demonstrated no invasion of submucosal tissue. Six months postoperatively he is doing well, with no evidence of recurrence. Cytoscopy has been negative and will be continued at 3- to 6-month intervals.

Clinical Pearls

1. A filling defect in the kidney can be caused by a stone, tumor, blood clot, fungus ball, sloughed papillae, or vascular impression.
2. Cystoscopy is necessary to rule out bladder neoplasia.
3. The gold-standard treatment is nephroureterectomy with resection of a bladder cuff.

REFERENCES

1. McDougall EM, Clayman RV, Elashry O: Laparascopic nephroureterectomy for upper tract transitional cell cancer: The Washington University experience. J Urol 154(3):975–997, 1995.
2. Tawfiek ER, Bagley DH: Upper-tract transitional cell carcinoma. Urology 50(3):321–329, 1997.
3. Jarrett TW: Endoscopic management of upper urinary TCC. Contemp Urol 10(6):60–73, 1998.
4. Messing EM, Catalona W: Urothelial tumors of the urinary tract. In Walsh PC, Retik AP, Stamey TA, Vaughan ED (eds): Cambell's Urology, 7th ed. Philadelphia, W.B. Saunders, 1998, pp 2327–2410.

PATIENT 18

A 53-year-old man with initial hematuria

A 53-year-old man presents with a complaint of blood in his urine. He states that he sees blood with the onset of urination, but that it clears while voiding. He denies any dysuria, but does feel that his stream has weakened over the last several months.

Physical Examination: Vital signs: normal. Abdomen: soft; no palpable inguinal adenopathy. Genitalia: testes descended bilaterally, no evidence of lesions; mildly tender, palpable mass in bulbous urethra. Rectum: 30-gram, smooth prostate.

Laboratory Findings: Urinalysis: negative for leukocyte esterase and nitrites. RBC 5–10/hpf, WBC 0–2/hpf; no bacteria. Serum electrolytes and complete blood count: normal. Prostate specific antigen: 1 (normal 1–4).

Question: What diagnostic studies are indicated?

Answer: Studies of the upper and lower urinary tract, including intravenous urogram and cysto-urethroscopy

Discussion: Urethral carcinoma is a rare disease in men, with approximately 600 cases reported. The etiology is unclear, but urethral stricture, venereal disease, and urethritis have been associated with urethral carcinoma. Unlike transitional cell carcinoma of the bladder and upper tracts, aromatic amines, cigarette smoking, and analgesic abuse have not been found to be associated with urethral carcinoma.

Human papilloma virus (HPV) previously has been associated with squamous papillomas of the urethra. Weiner and associates demonstrated an association between HPV-16 and squamous cell carcinoma of the male urethra. Their data supports HPV-16 as a probable etiologic effector in squamous cell carcinoma of the male urethra.

Signs and symptoms can be similar to those of urethral stricture. Patients may present with a palpable urethral mass, obstructive voiding symptoms, perineal pain, bleeding urethral fistula, or abscess.

The diagnosis is made by urethroscopy and biopsy. Often, a diagnosis of urethra stricture is made. Frequent dilatations, excessive bleeding after dilatation, or a friable necrotic mass should raise the index of suspicion. Needle biopsy or transurethral resection are required for diagnosis. Voided urine cytology also may be helpful.

Several staging systems have been reported. Ray and associates report a system similar to bladder cancer staging. The more recent TNM (tumor node metastasis) system is based on depth of invasion of the primary tumor, presence or absence of regional lymph node involvement, and presence or absence of distant metastasis. Staging requires bimanual examination, cystourethroscopy, and palpation of the inguinal nodes.

Surgical excision is the primary mode of treatment for carcinoma of the male urethra. Anterior urethral carcinoma makes up approximately 39% of all urethral carcinomas, and it responds especially well to surgical intervention and has a better prognosis in general. Lesions confined to the lamina propria can be treated with transurethral resection or open resection with primary anastomosis. Neodymium YAG laser also has been used with success. More invasive lesions require partial or total penectomy with or without emasculation to achieve a 2-centimeter free margin. Inguinal node dissection is indicated only in the presence of adenopathy or positive biopsy.

Proximal or bulbomembranous urethral carcinoma comprises approximately 54% of total cases. These cancers are commonly found at higher stages and have a poor prognosis. Superficial lesions are treated with transurethral resection or open resection with primary anastomosis. Extensive local disease requires wide radial resection. Radical cystoprostatectomy, pelvic lymphadenectomy, and total penectomy usually are required. Pubic rami resection may be required to improve the margin of resection and local control. Prophylactic inguinal node dissection does not improve survival. Regardless of treatment, chances of survival with carcinoma of the bulbomembranous urethra are poor.

In the present patient, intravenous urogram results were normal. However, cystourethroscopy revealed a friable, necrotic mass in the bulbomembranous urethra. Transurethral biopsy was performed, and the mass was determined to be a squamous cell carcinoma. Despite radical therapy, the patient died 24 months after presentation.

Clinical Pearls

1. When discussing urethral carcinoma, the bulbous urethra is considered in the posterior segment along with the conventional prostatic and membranous urethra.

2. The bulbomembranous urethra is the most common site of stricture and tumor.

3. Surgical excision is the primary mode of therapy for localized tumors. The extent of excision depends on location and depth of invasion.

REFERENCES
1. Weiner JS, Liu ET, Walther PJ: Oncogenic human papilloma virusType 16 is associated with squamous cell cancer of the male urethra. Cancer Res 52:5018, 1992.
2. Poore RE, McCullough DL: Urethral carcinoma. In Gillenwater JY, Grayhack JT, Howards SS, Duckett JW: Adult and Pediatric Urology. St. Louis, Mosby, 1996, pp 1837–1852.
3. Jordan GH, Schlossberg SM, Devine CJ: Surgery of the penis and urethra. In Walsh PC, Retik AB, Vaughan ED, Wein AJ (eds): Campbell's Urology. 7th ed. Philadelphia, W.B. Saunders, 1998, pp 3316–3394.
4. Davis JW, Schellhammer PF, Schlossberg SM: Conservative surgical therapy for penile and urethral carcinoma. Urology 53(2):386–392, 1999.

PATIENT 19

A 58-year-old man with a prostate nodule

A 58-year-old man presents to the urology clinic for evaluation of a prostatic nodule. He was seen initially by his primary care physician, who detected the nodule and also ordered a serum prostate specific antigen (PSA) test. The patient has not received any previous urologic evaluation. He denies obstructive and irritative voiding symptoms and has not experienced hematuria or urinary tract infection in the past. He has hypertension as well as noninsulin-dependent diabetes mellitus.

Physical Examination: General: moderately obese. Blood pressure 138/84, heart rate 70. Abdomen: obese, soft, and nontender. Genitalia: normal circumcised phallus; testes normal. Digital rectal exam: 40-gram prostate (2+) with nodule at right lateral apex; nodule 1-centimeter, firm, and nontender.

Laboratory Findings: Serum PSA: 7 ng/ml. Transrectal ultrasound-guided biopsy with sextant- and lesion-directed biopsies of the prostate: Gleason sum 3 + 3 adenocarcinoma in single biopsy core from right side; other core biopsies negative for cancer.

Questions: What is your diagnosis? Is further evaluation required?

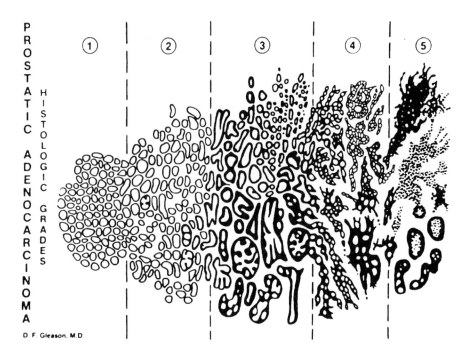

PROSTATIC ADENOCARCINOMA

HISTOLOGIC GRADES

D. F. Gleason, M.D.

Diagnosis: T2A adenocarcinoma

Discussion: The patient currently has disease localized to one side of the prostate. Further evaluation can at times include bone scan and pelvic lymphadenectomy. Bone scans are useful in detecting bone metastasis. However, in an asymptomatic patient with PSA less than 10 ng/ml, there is little chance of demonstrating bone metastasis. Bilateral obturator/pelvic lymphadenectomy often is performed to evaluate the possibility of regional metastasis. As with bone scans, the need for lymphadenectomy has become more focused by using PSA values and information obtained on prostate biopsy. Recent studies have shown that lymph node dissection in patients with PSA less than 10 ng/ml and well to moderately well differentiated cancers (Gleason sum < 7) may be unnecessary. Thus, neither lymphadenectomy nor bone scan are indicated in this patient.

This patient has a clinical stage T2A adenocarcinoma by the TNM classification system. T2A lesions are palpable tumors confined within the prostate that involve half a lobe or less. The natural history of the prostate cancer is that of a slow-growing tumor. The decision to treat should consider the patient's actuarial survival as well as comorbid conditions. If the patient does not have an estimated 10-year life expectancy, curative therapy generally is not recommended.

Treatment options for localized prostate cancer include radical prostatectomy and external beam radiation. Interstitial radiotherapy and cryotherapy are in the stages of development and evaluation. Their results have not reached the period of followup obtained with radical surgery and external beam radiation.

Radical prostatectomy and external beam radiation offer definitive treatment for localized disease. Statistics regarding local control and cause-specific survival vary greatly between and within each treatment modality. Fifteen year cause-specific survival ranges from 52–82% for radiation and radical prostatectomy; however, these statistics are difficult to compare due to patient selection bias. More recent studies using comparable patients and followup times demonstrate good short-term but limited long-term results with radiation therapy. Five-year survival without biochemical evidence of disease (bNED) occurred in 60–69% of patients, versus 83% for external radiation and radical prostatectomy, respectively. The 10-year bNED survival was 20–40% versus 47–70%; 15-year bNED survival was 17–46% versus 40–75%, respectively. Certainly further studies will be needed to compare these treatment modalities. It is likely that both radical prostatectomy and external beam radiation will continue to have a role in the treatment of localized prostate cancer.

In the present patient, radical prostatectomy and external beam radiation achieved good short-term success, with bNED at 3 years. He will be followed closely.

Clinical Pearls

1. Bone scans are not indicated in asymptomatic patients with PSA less than 10 ng/ml.
2. Lymphadenectomy may be unnecessary with PSA less than 10 ng/ml.
3. External beam radiation and radical prostatectomy are currently accepted definitive treatments for localized prostate cancer.

REFERENCES
1. Zincke H, et al: Long-term (15 years) results after radical prostatectomy for clinically localized (stage T2c or lower) prostate cancer. J Urol 152(5 Pt 2):1850–1857, 1994.
2. Sullivan LD, Rabbani F: Should we reconsider the indications for ileo-obturator node dissection with localized prostate cancer? Br J Urol 75(1):33–37, 1995.
3. Goluboff ET, Benson MC: External beam radiation therapy does not offer long-term control of prostate cancer. Urol Clin North Am 23(4):617–621, 1996.

PATIENT 20

An 83-year-old man with a prostate nodule

An 83-year-old certified public accountant with mild obstructive voiding symptoms presents for evaluation of a prostate nodule detected during a community prostate cancer screening session. The patient denies constitutional symptoms, including bone pain. He is otherwise healthy, is taking no medications, and has no family history of prostate cancer. His parents lived to ages 88 and 91.

Physical Examination: Temperature 37°; heart rate 84; blood pressure 110/70. Genitalia: penis circumcised with no lesions; testes descended bilaterally with no masses or nodules, nontender to palpation; prostate 1+ in size with well-circumscribed, nontender nodule approximately 0.5 centimeter in diameter at right apex.

Laboratory Findings: Urine dipstick: nitrite negative, leukocyte esterase negative, heme 1+. Microscopic urinalysis: RBC 0–2/hpf, WBC 0–2/hpf. Urine cultures: negative. Prostate specific antigen (PSA): 7 ng/ml.

Question: What is the most likely diagnosis?

Diagnosis: Prostate cancer

Discussion: Prostatitis may be acute or chronic. In **acute prostatitis**, signs and symptoms are consistent with inflammation and/or infection of the prostate gland and include fever, dysuria, perineal pain, urinary frequency, and positive urine cultures. Clinically, the prostate is tender and boggy. The patient with **chronic prostatitis** typically presents with a history of persistent bacterial infections despite prolonged antibiotic therapy. These patients may have prostatic calculi-containing bacteria serving as a potential source of reinfection. PSA may rise with prostatitis, but usually normalizes following antibiotics. Other forms of prostatitis include: nonspecific granulomatis prostatitis, tuberculous prostatitis, mycotic prostatitis, parasitic prostatitis, and gonococcal prostatitis.

The differential diagnosis includes **benign prostatic hypertrophy** (BPH), prostatitis, and carcinoma of the prostate. A patient with BPH often presents with symptoms consistent with bladder outlet obstruction. On physical exam the prostate is variably enlarged, with a rubbery consistency. A discrete prostate nodule is an unlikely finding in the patient with only BPH.

The diagnosis typically is made by screening digital rectal exam and PSA. If abnormalities in one or both exist, then transrectal ultrasound and biopsy of the prostate are performed. A tissue sample is obtained to confirm the diagnosis and establish a tumor grade. A PSA floor of 4.0 ng/ml is an effective threshold to maximize detection and to minimize unnecessary biopsies.

Management options for localized prostate cancer should focus on the natural history of disease progression and survivability. Studies have found that disease-specific survival for localized disease at 10 years was 83% for deferred therapy, 93% for radical prostatectomy, and 62% for external radiotherapy. In patients over age 70, invasive treatment may be harmful, and associated morbidity related to treatment must be considered. Furthermore, death from untreated localized prostate cancer occurs only after a protracted course. Therefore, it generally is believed that there is no need to treat localized prostate cancer in patients with limited life spans.

In the present patient, transrectal ultrasound and biopsy were presented as diagnostic options, with the understanding that a positive biopsy would probably not result in aggressive treatment. After declining transrectal ultrasound and biopsy, yearly physical exams and PSA evaluations were performed. Though his PSA continued to rise slowly to 27 ng/ml, he did not complain of obstructive voiding or constitutional symptoms. The patient remained active, working two days a week until his death at age 89 of nondisease-related causes.

Clinical Pearls

1. Treatment for localized prostate cancer should focus on the natural history of disease progression.

2. In patients over age 70, invasive treatment may be harmful and the associated morbidity of treatment must be considered.

3. Death from localized prostate cancer usually occurs only after a protracted course.

4. There is no need to aggressively treat localized prostate cancer in men with limited lifespans.

REFERENCES
1. Adolfsson J, Steineck G, Whitmore WF Jr: Results of the management of palpable clinically localized prostate cancer. Cancer 72:43–55, 1993.
2. Albertson PC, Fryback DG, Storer BE, et al: Long-term survival among men conservatively treated for localized prostate cancer. JAMA 274:626, 1995.
3. Fowler FJ Jr, Barry MS, Lu-Yao G, et al: The effects of radical prostatectomy for prostate cancer on patient quality of life: Results from a Medicare survey. Urology 45:1007–1015, 1995.
4. Meares FM Jr: Prostatitis and related disorders. In Walsh PC, Retik AB, Vaughan AD Jr, Wein AJ (eds): Campbell's Urology, 7th ed. Philadelphia, W.B. Saunders, 1998, pp 615–630.
5. Walsh PC: The natural history of localized prostate cancer: A guide to therapy. In Walsh PC, Retik AB, Vaughan AD Jr, Wein AJ (eds): Campbell's Urology, 7th ed. Philadelphia, W.B. Saunders, 1998, pp 2539–2546.

PATIENT 21

A 63-year-old man with a gradual rise in prostate specific antigen over 3 years

A 63-year-old man is seen by his urologist for his annual digital rectal exam and prostate specific antigen (PSA) test. In the past he has had normal digital rectal exams. Three years ago his PSA was 0.5 ng/ml; 2 years ago it was 1.0 ng/ml; last year it was 2.0 ng/ml. He denies any new back, bone, or joint pains and has only mild obstructive voiding symptoms. He takes no other medication and is otherwise in good health.

Physical Examination: Vital signs: normal. Abdomen: soft, without palpable masses or adenopathy. Genitalia: normal. Digital rectal exam: 30-gram prostate without nodularity or induration.

Laboratory Findings: PSA 2 weeks prior: 3.0 ng/ml.

Question: Is this patient's slowly rising PSA indicative of a neoplasm?

Answer: Possibly, yes

Discussion: Prostate-specific antigen is believed to be the single test with the highest positive prediction value for cancer. Used in conjunction with a digital rectal examination, PSA increases the detection of prostate cancer and organ-confined disease. However, the test has limitations.

Serum PSA results do not differentiate between elevations secondary to malignancy and benign prostatic hyperplasia (BPH). Multiple investigations have focused on methods, such as PSA density, age-specific PSA, free/total PSA, and PSA velocity, to improve this distinguishing capability. PSA velocity is a measure of the change in PSA over time. PSA velocity has high specificity because few men (less than 5%) without prostate cancer have a **PSA velocity** indicating the presence of cancer.

Substantial variability in serum PSA can occur between repeat PSA measurements in the presence or absence of prostate cancer. Short-term changes are due primarily to physiologic variation. It has been shown that among individuals, PSA variability is 46–49% of the mean of multiple PSA measures in 95% of men. Thus, short-term changes cannot be used alone to discriminate between men with and without prostate cancer. The variability in PSA can be corrected by using elapsed time between measurements or PSA velocity.

Carter and associates showed that an increase in PSA greater than 0.75 ng/ml per year was a specific marker for prostate cancer. Seventy-two percent of men with prostate cancer had a PSA velocity of 0.75 ng/ml or more per year, whereas only 5% of men without prostate cancer had a PSA velocity above 0.75 ng/ml per year.

The minimum length of time over which PSA velocity is useful is 1.5–2 years. Kadmon showed that 12.5% of patients had a single PSA velocity greater than 0.75 ng/ml per year, but only 0.4% had PSA velocity greater than 0.75 ng/ml per year evaluated over a 2-year period. It also appears that three PSA values are needed for optimal accuracy of PSA velocity in evaluation for prostate cancer.

The present patient has a PSA velocity of 0.83 ng/ml per year over 3 years, with four separate PSA values. Although his PSA is in the "normal" range, prostate biopsy should be considered. The rate of PSA increase should make the clinician suspicious of a prostatic neoplasm.

Clinical Pearls

1. Substantial variability in serum PSA can occur between measurements in men with and without prostate cancer.

2. In PSA velocity adjusted over a 1.5- to 2-year period, less than 5% of men without prostate cancer will have a PSA velocity greater than 0.75 ng/ml per year, and 70% with prostate cancer will have a PSA velocity of 0.75 ng/ml or greater per year.

3. Three PSA values are needed to optimize PSA velocity specificity.

4. PSA velocity is a specific marker for prostate cancer.

REFERENCES

1. Carter HB, Pearson JD, Metter JE, et al: Longitudinal evaluation of prostate-specific antigen levels in men with and without prostate disease. JAMA 267:2215–2220, 1992.
2. Carter HB, Pearson JD, Waclawiw Z, et al: Prostate-specific antigen variability in men without prostate cancer: The effect of sampling interval and number of repeat measurements on prostate-specific antigen velocity. Urology 45:591–596, 1995.
3. Kadmon D, Weinberb AD, Williams RH, et al: Pitfalls in interpreting prostate specific antigen velocity. J Urol 155:1655–1657, 1996.
4. Komatsu K, Wehner N, Prestigiacomo AF, et al: Physiologic (intraindividual) variation of serum prostate specific antigen in 814 men from a screening population. Urology 47:343–346, 1996.
5. Carter HB, Partin AW: Diagnosis and staging of prostate cancer. In Walsh PC, Retik AB, Vaughan ED, Wein AJ (eds): Campbell's Urology, 7th ed. Philadelphia, W.B. Saunders, 1998, pp 2519–2537.

PATIENT 22

A 78-year-old man with a prostate nodule and bone pain

A 78-year-old man presents to the clinician with a 1-month history of worsening lower back and lower extremity pain. Nonsteroidal anti-inflammatory medications no longer afford him symptomatic relief. He has noticed a recent 15-pound weight loss, as well as a slowing of his urinary stream and worsening nocturia over the past several months.

Physical Examination: Vital signs: normal. Cardiac: normal. Abdomen: benign. Neurologic: normal. Genitalia: penis uncircumcised without lesions or discharges; testes bilaterally descended without masses; large, hard nodule in prostate on right, replacing entire lobe and extending into ipsilateral seminal vesicle.

Laboratory Findings: WBC 5200/µl, Hct 28%. Creatinine 1.2 mg/dl, alkaline phosphatase 1200 IU/L, prostate specific antigen (PSA) 850 ng/dl, prostatic acid phosphatase (tartrate inhibited) 12.6 IU/L. Urinalysis: negative for WBCs, RBCs, and bacteria. Transrectally obtained biopsy of prostate: 6/6 cores positive for adenocarcinoma, Gleason grade 7. Radionuclide bone scan: diffuse uptake of radiopharmaceutical in skeleton, suggesting metastatic disease (see figure).

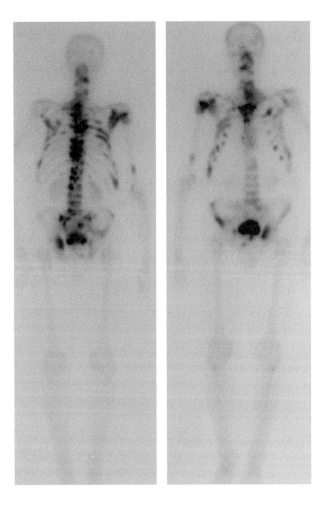

Diagnosis: Adenocarcinoma of the prostate, metastatic to bone

Discussion: Adenocarcinoma of the prostate (ACaP) is the most common solid tumor in males and is the second leading cause of cancer-specific death. Much controversy has arisen in recent years regarding the optimal means of treating the localized form of the disease, with observation, surgery, and radiation each having its proponents. However, metastatic ACaP requires prompt diagnosis and treatment because it is a debilitating disease. Moreover, it often responds dramatically to simple treatments.

PSA, a kallikrein glycoprotein secreted almost exclusively by the prostate, is a sensitive marker for prostate cancer, if elevated. PSA has largely supplanted acid phosphatase as a marker for ACaP, but an elevated acid phosphatase can be an important indicator of metastases. As the most common site for metastatic deposits in ACaP is bone, a radionuclide bone scan remains the most important radiographic examination.

The standard treatment for prostate cancer for the past half-century has been, and remains, hormonal ablation. Approximately 75% of metastatic prostate cancer is hormonally dependent for proliferation. The withdrawal of androgens results in cellular apoptosis and disease regression. Hormonally ablative regimens almost invariably fail eventually, however, because of the emergence of hormonally refractory cells. Nonetheless, androgen ablation can extend life and improve its quality for the patient.

Several options currently are employed for hormonal ablation therapy in patients with metastatic prostate cancer. Surgical orchiectomy is the simplest and results in the fastest drop in serum testosterone. However, many men are reluctant to undergo this procedure; so-called chemical castrating agents can be used instead. These drugs interrupt the hypothalamic-pituitary-gonadal axis at various steps. Goserelin and leuprolide are luteinizing hormone-releasing hormone (LHRH) analogues that interrupt the normal pulsatile release of LHRH from the hypothalamus to the anterior pituitary gland, thereby shutting the entire axis down at this level. Diethylstilbesterol (DES) and other estrogen-like substances work by inhibiting the release of LH at the level of the pituitary by negative feedback. Any of these treatments is equally effective, and the specific therapy should be individualized to the patient. Common side effects include hot flashes and loss of libido. DES increases the risk of thromboembolic phenomena and should be used with caution.

In the present patient, physical examination results are typical of a large, extensive tumor of the prostate. This finding, in combination with the patient's description of worsening lower back pain and urinary symptoms, alerts the physician to the possibility of metastatic ACaP. The Gleason score of this tumor is relatively high, suggesting an aggressive disease. Radiographic evidence of bony metastases marks the disease as stage D2 by the TNM system. The metastases explains the elevated alkaline phosphatase and also might explain the low hematocrit if the bone marrow is involved.

The patient underwent an uneventful orchiectomy. His pain improved within 24 hours of the procedure. One month later, his PSA, alkaline phosphatase, and prostatic acid phosphatase were almost normal, and he had regained 8 pounds of his 15-pound loss. His urinary symptoms have begun to improve.

Clinical Pearls

1. Patients with prostatic nodules, lower urinary tract symptoms, and bone pain may have metastatic adenocarcinoma of the prostate.
2. Hormonal ablation remains the cornerstone of treatment for metastatic ACaP and should be instituted as soon as possible to treat the symptomatic patient.

REFERENCE
Garnick MB: Hormonal therapy in the management of prostate cancer: From Huggins to the present. Urology 49(3a):5–14, 1997.

PATIENT 23

A 46-year-old man with abdominal pain and hematuria

A 46-year-old man with hypertension presents with a 2-month history of right abdominal pain and intermittent gross hematuria. He denies any prior history of trauma or urolithiasis. He is taking a calcium channel-blocker for hypertension. The remainder of his medical history is unremarkable.

Physical Examination: Blood pressure 160/82; pulse 78. Abdomen: palpable right abdominal mass inferior to liver edge. Genitalia: normal. Prostate: normal.

Laboratory Findings: CBC: normal. Serum creatinine: 1.1 mg/dl. Urinalysis: loaded RBC, no WBC, no granular casts, no bacteria. Urinary cytology: negative. Intravenous urogram: large right renal mass displacing renal collecting system. Computed tomographic (CT) scan of abdomen: see figure.

Question: What is the most likely diagnosis?

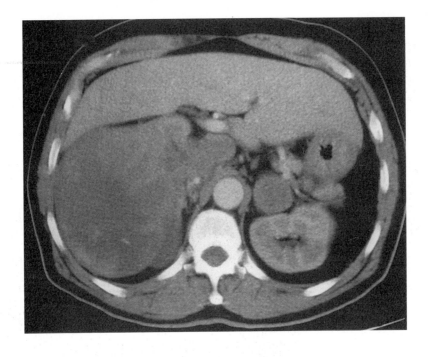

Diagnosis: Renal cell carcinoma with invasion of the right renal vein and vena cava

Discussion: Renal cell carcinoma (RCC) is a relatively rare tumor, accounting for approximately 3% of adult malignancies. It is more common in males than females (2:1 ratio) and occurs predominantly in adults 40–60 years of age.

Renal cell carcinomas arise from the proximal convoluted tubule. The etiology generally is unclear; however, there appears to be a link with cigarette smoking. Alterations in the short arm of chromosome 3, most commonly seen in nonfamilial RCC, led to studies of the familial form of renal cancer associated with von Hippel-Lindau (VHL) disease with the presumption that both may involve the same gene. Von Hippel-Lindau disease is a rare familial cancer syndrome in which affected individuals develop tumors in various locations, including the kidneys. Renal cell carcinomas associated with VHL disease are known to metastasize and are responsible for nearly 40% of VHL disease deaths when not recognized and treated early.

RCC typically is unilateral, but bilateral involvement has been reported in 2% of cases. The tumors classically have been grouped into four histologic types: clear cell, granular cell, tubulopapillary, and sarcomatoid. The clear cell variant is the most common and accounts for over 80% of these neoplasms. The sarcomatoid variant is a more aggressive tumor and usually portends a poor prognosis. A new type—the chromophobe type—appears to be associated with improved survival.

Renal cell carcinomas present in a variety of ways. The classic triad of pain, hematuria, and flank mass is considered pathognomonic, but is found in few patients and usually indicates advanced disease. Hematuria is the most common presenting sign, occurring in 60% of patients. Pain, weight loss, fever, varicocele, and hypertension also may occur. Patients may present with a variety of paraneoplastic syndromes or with nonmetastatic hepatic dysfunction (known as Staufer syndrome).

The diagnosis of RCC usually is based on findings of various radiographic studies. Intravenous urography is the most commonly used initial modality. Ultrasonography is useful in differentiating solid masses from cystic masses. Indeterminate renal masses detected by ultrasound should be further evaluated with abdominal CT scanning. CT is the method of choice for detecting and staging RCC. Magnetic resonance imaging (MRI) is useful for patients with intravenous contrast allergies. Both CT and MRI can detect tumor extension into the renal vein and inferior vena cava as well as assess for adenopathy. Sometimes, venacavography is necessary to identify tumor thrombi within the vena cava.

The most commonly used staging systems for RCC are the Robson and the tumor, node, and metastases (TNM) classifications. The two are compared below:

Staging of Renal Cell Carcinoma

	Robson	TNM
Small tumor, confined to capsule	I	T1
Large tumor, confined to capsule	I	T2
Extension into fat or ipsilateral adrenal	II	T3a
Renal vein involvement	IIIa	T3b
Renal vein and inferior vena cava	IIIa	T3c
Inferior vena cava above diaphragm	IIIa	T4b
Single ipsilateral node	IIIb	N1
Multiple regional, contralateral, or bilateral nodes	IIIb	N2
Fixed regional nodes	IIIb	N3
Juxtaregional nodes	IIIb	N4
Combination IIIa and IIIb	IIIc	T3,4 N1–4
Spread to adjacent organs (except adrenal)	IVa	T4a
Distant metastases	IVb	M1

Surgical removal of the kidney is the only effective treatment for localized RCC. Radical nephrectomy is the treatment of choice for Stage I, II, and some Stage III tumors. For patients with bilateral renal tumors or a tumor in a solitary kidney, nephron-sparing surgery is indicated.

The potential for RCC to invade the renal veins and extend into the main renal vein has been well documented. Continued growth of the thrombus into the vena cava occurs in a small number of patients, usually without direct invasion of the vessel. In the past, vena caval extension was felt to be a sign of poor prognosis, with little chance for cure. Five-year survival rates of 50–70% have been reported following complete surgical excision in patients with nonmetastatic RCC and vena caval involvement. The current literature indicates that excision of renal cell carcinomas with vena caval extension remains the treatment of choice and can be performed safely, even with extension into the right atrium. When radical nephrectomy with removal of a thrombus in the inferior vena cava is performed, the vena cava above the thrombus must be controlled to prevent intraoperative embolization of tumor thrombi. For supradiaphragmatic thrombi, adjunctive cardiopulmonary bypass with deep hypothermic circulatory arrest sometimes is necessary for complete surgical removal.

In the present patient, CT scanning confirmed pulmonary metastases and determined the stage to be TNM IIIa (Robson T3c). His hematuria worsened, and his hematocrit decreased. Palliative nephrectomy was performed. The patient had an uneventful postoperative course and was discharged on postoperative day number 7. His hematocrit was corrected with blood products and remained stable after surgery. He suffered no further episodes of hematuria.

Clinical Pearls

1. The most common presenting signs and symptoms of renal cell carcinoma are hematuria, flank or abdominal pain, and a palpable mass.
2. The clear cell variant of RCC is the most common histologic type and accounts for over 80% of these neoplasms.
3. Assessment of the inferior vena cava for presence of tumor thrombus in a patient with RCC is done with CT, MRI, and/or venacavography.
4. The 5-year survival rate in patients with nonmetastatic RCC and inferior vena cava involvement is 50–70% following complete surgical excision.

REFERENCES
1. Skinner DG, Pritchett TR, Lieskovsky G, et al: Vena caval involvement by renal cell carcinoma. Ann Surg 201(3):387–394, 1989.
2. Novick AC, Kaye MC, Cosgrove DM, et al: Experience with cardiopulmonary bypass and deep hypothermic circulatory arrest in the management of retroperitoneal tumors with large vena caval thrombi. Ann Surg 212(4):472–477, 1990.
3. Jennings SB, Linehan WM: Renal, perirenal, and ureteral neoplasms. In Gillenwater JY, Grayhack JT, Howards SS, Duckett JW (eds): Adult and Pediatric Urology, 3rd ed. St. Louis, Mosby, 1996.

PATIENT 24

A 68-year-old woman with a urethral mass

A 68-year-old woman presented with a painless mass at the urethral meatus. She reported a history of urinary frequency, but denied any dysuria, hematuria, or urinary tract infection.

Physical Examination: Blood pressure 110/74; pulse 82. Abdomen: soft, without masses or tenderness. Genitalia: 2.0-centimeter diameter, red, polyploid mass located at urethral meatus (see figure).

Laboratory Findings: CBC and sequential multiple analysis-7: normal. Urinalysis: RBC 2–3/hpf, WBC 0–2/hpf; no bacteria; leukocyte esterase and nitrite negative.

Question: What is the most likely diagnosis?

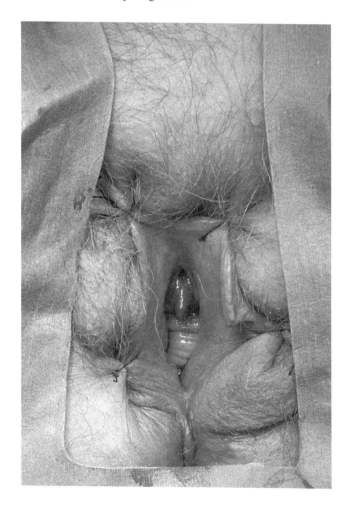

Diagnosis: Urethral caruncle

Discussion: Urethral caruncle is a clinical term used to describe a small, polyploid lesion arising from the posterior wall at or near the meatus. Urethral caruncle was first described by Samuel Sharp in 1750. The lesion appears as dusky red in color; ranges in size from 1–2 millimeters to 1–2 centimeters; may be sessile or pedunculated; and may appear ulcerated, friable, or hemorrhagic. Recurrence typically is high.

It is postulated that urethral caruncle is the end result of subepithelial or periurethral inflammation and scarring. This scarring is caused by inflammation of the paraurethral (Skene's) ducts or other sources of chronic inflammation and irritation. Histologically, urethral caruncles are composed of loose vascular connective tissue covered by squamous or transitional cell epithelium. Their location at or near the urethral meatus predisposes them to inflammation, and the subsequent vascular granulation tissue may histologically appear as a pyogenic granuloma, an angioma, or a vascular polyp. Rarely, a carcinoma, sarcoma, or lymphoma may be mistakenly identified as a caruncle.

The symptoms of urethral caruncle include: painful urination, bleeding, urinary frequency and urgency, and the appearance of a mass. The degree of impairment varies, as these lesions may be asymptomatic or severely incapacitating. Affected women range in age from 40–70 years, with caruncles most commonly occurring in postmenopausal and multiparous women.

The successful treatment of urethral caruncle depends upon removal of the scar tissue, typically accomplished via surgical excision. Excision using electrocautery with fulguration of the base has been reported to be superior to simple excisional methods. Recurrence may be the result of failure to excise all scar tissue as well as the urethral caruncle.

The present patient underwent successful excision of the urethral caruncle and scar tissue. Pathology revealed an inflammatory mass with evidence of granulation tissue. There was no evidence of malignant tissue.

Clinical Pearls

1. Urethral caruncle is believed to result from subepithelial or periurethral inflammation and scarring.

2. Successful treatment of urethral caruncle depends upon successful removal of the scar tissue along with the caruncle.

3. A carcinoma, sarcoma, or malignant lymphoma may mimic urethral caruncle.

REFERENCES
1. Becker LE: Urethral caruncle: A herald lesion for distal urethral stenosis? J Natl Med Assoc 67(3):228–230, 1975.
2. Bolduan JP, Farah RN: Primary urethral neoplasms: Review of 30 cases. J Urol 125:198–200, 1981.
3. Tanagho EA: Disorders of the female urethra. In Tanagho EA, McAninch JW (eds): Smith's General Urology, 14th ed. Norwalk, Appleton & Lange, 1995.
4. Nichols DH, Randall CL: Minor and ambulatory surgery. In Mitchell CW (ed): Vaginal Surgery, 4th ed. Baltimore, Williams & Wilkins, 1996.

PATIENT 25

A 61-year-old man with flank pain following resection of the sigmoid colon

A 61-year-old man with a history of Dukes B1 colon cancer presents with complaints of urinary incontinence and bilateral flank pain. He is 3 months status post sigmoid colectomy.

Physical Examination: Blood pressure 142/78; pulse 80. Abdomen: soft, nontender, no palpable masses. Extremities: minimal left flank tenderness, no right flank tenderness. Genitalia: normal. Prostate: 20 grams, no nodules.

Laboratory Findings: CBC: normal. BUN 28 mg/dl, creatinine 2.0 mg/dl. Urinalysis: negative. Intravenous urogram: delayed image (see figure).

Question: What is your diagnosis?

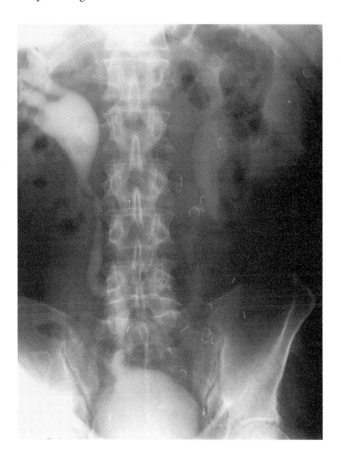

Diagnosis: Iatrogenic ureteral injury related to colon resection

Discussion: Ureteral injury is a potential complication of abdominal or pelvic surgery, with a reported incidence of 0.5%–1%. If unrecognized, ureteral injuries may result in sepsis and loss of renal function. Gynecologic surgery traditionally has accounted for more than 50% of all injuries, while general surgical (5–15%) and urological (30%) procedures make up the rest. Recently, however, an increase has been reported in urological-related injuries.

Iatrogenic ureteral injuries may result from complete or partial ligation by a suture; inadvertent application of hemostatic clamps; complete or partial transection; or excision of a segment of ureter—all of which may compromise the ureteral blood supply, resulting in necrosis and fistula formation. The most frequent injuries seem to be complete ligation and complete transection.

The symptoms associated with injury to the ureter depend upon whether the injury is unilateral or bilateral, the degree of obstruction that is created, the time interval that has occurred since the injury, and the presence of urinary extravasation. A thorough history usually elicits symptoms indicative of the diagnosis. In the initial postoperative period, mild flank pain and tenderness may be overshadowed by incisional pain or abdominal distension related to ileus. The patient may or may not be febrile. If the injury is unilateral, renal function and urinary output may be unaffected. Complete bilateral ureteral occlusion, however, presents with anuria.

More pronounced symptoms occur with infection, which typically elicits pain, fever, abdominal distension, and possibly sepsis. Urinary extravasation may result in fistulas to the vagina, perineum, skin, or bowel. If a fistula is suspected, cystoscopy and retrograde pyelography or intravenous urography should be performed to confirm the diagnosis. When symptoms are absent or minimal, the diagnosis of ureteral injury becomes quite difficult and may go unrecognized for several months.

Prompt recognition of ureteral injuries at the time of occurrence and immediate surgical repair results in fewer complications and decreased loss of renal units. Injuries detected postoperatively require more procedures to repair the ureter. The treatment of ureteral injuries is influenced by the length of time since the injury, the site and type of injury, the presence of a unilateral or a bilateral injury, and the general health of the patient. Surgical options for repair range from simple urinary diversion with or without ureteral stenting to reanastomosis, reimplantation, or nephrectomy.

In the present patient, the intravenous urogram revealed right hydroureteronephrosis, with minimal faint visualization of the left kidney and ureter. He was determined to have bilateral distal ureteral obstruction with relatively diminished renal function on the left. Urinary diversion with ureteral stenting was performed bilaterally initially. The right kidney maintained adequate function; however, the left kidney eventually deteriorated to minimal function. The patient ultimately sustained left pyohydronephrosis and underwent left nephrectomy, with successful repair of his ureteral injury.

Clinical Pearls

1. Recognition of iatrogenic ureteral injury at the time of surgery results in fewer complications and decreased loss of renal units.

2. Iatrogenic ureteral injuries usually occur secondary to gynecological (50%), general surgical (5–15%), or urological (30%) procedures.

REFERENCES

1. Higgins CC: Ureteral injuries during surgery. JAMA 199(2):118–124, 1967.
2. Hughes ESR, McDermott FT, Polglase AL, Johnson WR: Ureteric damage in surgery for cancer of the large bowel. Dis Colon Rectum 27:293–295, 1984.
3. Selzman AA, Spirnak JP: Iatrogenic ureteral injuries: A 20-year experience in treating 165 injuries. J Urol 155:878–881, 1996.

PATIENT 26

A 37-year-old woman with microscopic hematuria

A 37-year-old female presents for evaluation of persistent microscopic hematuria over the last 3 months. She denies any pain or irritative voiding symptoms over this time period and has no other complaints. Her past medical history is significant for a urinary tract infection 1 year ago. She does not smoke and has no previous surgical history.

Physical Examination: Vital signs: normal. Abdomen: no masses or tenderness to palpation. Extremities: normal. Genitalia: normal.

Laboratory Findings: CBC, BUN, serum creatinine, and electrolytes: normal. Urinalysis: RBC 10–20/hpf, no WBC, no granular casts, no bacteria. Urine culture: negative. Intravenous pyelogram: see figure. Cystoscopy of bladder: normal.

Question: What is your diagnosis?

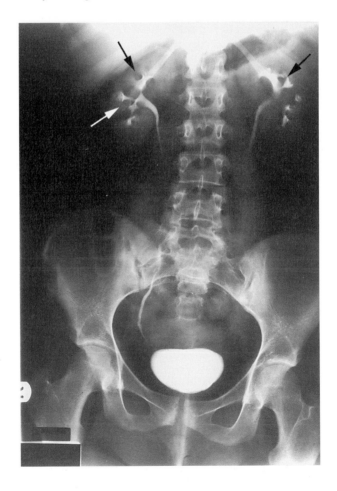

Diagnosis: Medullary sponge kidney

Discussion: Medullary sponge kidney (MSK) is a disease process of unknown pathogenesis that is diagnosed by excretory urography. The kidneys retain their reniform shape and tend to be bilaterally involved, with 1- to 5-mm medullary cysts. These cysts are dilated collecting ducts present at the papillary tips of the renal pyramids. The incidence of MSK ranges from 1 in 5000 to 1 in 20,000.

Patients with MSK typically are 20–50 years of age and present with symptoms that initiate an evaluation by intravenous urography. The most common presenting symptoms include renal colic (in 50–60% of patients), urinary tract infection (in 20–33%), and gross hematuria (in 10–18%). However, an uncertain number of patients go undiagnosed because they remain asymptomatic. Of the patients diagnosed with MSK, approximately 60% will pass calculi at some time in their life. Nephrocalcinosis occurs and can lead to stone formation and passage. Stones usually are composed of calcium phosphate. The cause of stone formation in MSK is unknown, but urinary stagnation in the dilated collecting ducts and defective urinary acidification may play roles. Also, one-third to one-half of patients with MSK have been found to have hypercalcemia.

The diagnosis of MSK is made on excretory urography by observing contrast medium stagnating in the dilated tubules in one or more renal papillae. The tubules appear as linear radiations arising from the calyces (see figure, *arrows*). Calculi located at the papillary tips and nephrocalcinosis may be identified on plain abdominal radiography.

Treatment for MSK is dependent on the disease complications, as some patients have an asymptomatic course. Urinary tract infections in patients with MSK respond well to antibiotics. Extracorporeal shock-wave lithotripsy is effective in the treatment of symptomatic stones in the collecting system, but is not effective in fragmenting ductal calcifications. Prevention of stone formation with increased fluid intake, thiazides, and inorganic phosphates can be attempted. The prognosis for patients with MSK also depends on the complications: it has been estimated that 10% of symptomatic patients have a poor long-term prognosis because of nephrolithiasis, sepsis, and renal failure.

The present patient remained asymptomatic with no further urinary tract infections, and is followed yearly with a plain abdominal radiograph and urinalysis.

Clinical Pearls

1. Calculi are passed by 60% of patients diagnosed with medullary sponge kidney.

2. Metabolic disorders accounting for nephrolithiasis are found less commonly in patients with stones and MSK than in patients with stones but no MSK.

3. Calcium phosphate stones are the most common stones found in patients with MSK, followed by calcium oxalate.

4. MSK is a disease process of unknown pathogenesis that is diagnosed by excretory urography.

REFERENCES

1. Kuiper JJ: Medullary sponge kidney. In Gardner KD Jr (ed): Cystic Diseases of the Kidney. New York, John Wiley & Sons, 1976.
2. Lippert MC: Renal cystic disease. In Gillenwater JY, Grayhack JT, Howards SS, Duckett JW (eds): Adult and Pediatric Urology, 3rd ed. St. Louis, Mosby, 1996.
3. Levine E, Hartman DS, Meilstrup JW, et al: Current concepts and controversies in imaging of renal cystic diseases. Urol Clin North Am 24(3):523–543, 1997.
4. Hsu TH, Streem SB: Metabolic abnormalities in patients with caliceal diverticular calculi. J Urol 160(5):1640–1642, 1998.

PATIENT 27

A 67-year-old woman with gross hematuria

A 67-year-old woman with hypertension experienced two episodes of gross, total, painless hematuria over the past 2 months. She has no prior history of calculi, flank injury, or bleeding disorders. Aside from smoking one pack of cigarettes a day for 40 years, the remainder of the patient's history is unremarkable.

Physical Examination: Pulse 80; blood pressure 155/80. Abdomen: no masses nor tenderness to palpation. Extremities: no flank masses. Genitalia: normal.

Laboratory Findings: CBC, BUN, serum creatinine, and electrolytes: normal. Urinalysis: loaded RBC, no WBC, no granular casts, no bacteria; atypical uroepithelial cells with rare papillary clusters on cytologic study. Intravenous urography: persistent filling defect in right renal pelvis. Cystoscopy: normal bladder. Right retrograde pyelogram: see figure.

Question: What is your diagnosis?

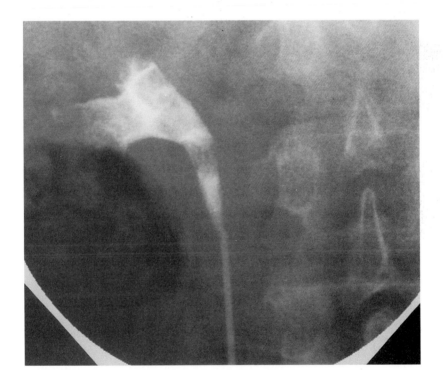

Diagnosis: Transitional cell carcinoma of the renal pelvis

Discussion: Transitional cell carcinoma (TCC) of the renal pelvis accounts for only 6–7% of all renal cancers and about 5% of all urothelial cancers. Of renal pelvic cancers, more than 90% are transitional cell carcinomas, while squamous cell and adenocarcinomas account for most of the remainder. The incidence of bilateral tumors is 2–5%, and approximately 30–50% of patients with renal pelvic TCC subsequently develop TCC of the bladder. Diagnosis of upper urinary tract urothelial cancers usually occurs in the sixth and seventh decades of life.

Factors that have been implicated in the etiology of renal pelvic cancers include occupational exposure to aniline and benzidine dyes, coal, coke, asphalt, and tar. Cigarette smoking and analgesic abuse with phenacetin are both established predisposing factors for the development of upper tract transitional cell carcinomas. Balkan nephropathy is associated with an increased incidence of upper urinary tract TCC found in patients from Bulgaria, Greece, Romania, and Yugoslavia. These lesions tend to be small, low grade, and superficial, and are bilateral in 10% of patients.

The most common presenting symptom of upper tract urothelial tumors is **gross hematuria**, which is seen in approximately 75% of patients. The presence of blood throughout urination and the passage of a vermiform clot suggest an upper tract source. Flank pain occurs in up to 30% of patients and can be dull if it is secondary to ureteral obstruction from the tumor or acute if due to blood clots. Irritative voiding symptoms occur in 5–10% of patients, and only 10% present with a flank mass due to hydronephrosis or a large tumor. Rarely, patients present with no symptoms, or with systemic symptoms of anorexia, weight loss, fatigue, and bone pain, representing metastatic disease.

The diagnosis usually is confirmed using a combination of intravenous urography, retrograde pyelography, and selective upper urinary tract cytology. On intravenous urography, approximately 50–75% of patients have an irregular filling defect that is in contact with the wall of the collecting system. In 10–30%, the tumor may cause nonvisualization or obstruction of the collecting system. Cystoscopy with retrograde pyelography is mandatory to rule out the presence of coexisting bladder tumors and to further evaluate the entire collecting system and ureter. Retrograde pyelography provides better visualization of the collecting system and has an overall 75% accuracy in establishing the diagnosis of urothelial cancer. Nonionic contrast is preferred for performing retrograde studies because hyperosmotic contrast may alter cytologic studies.

Computed tomography and ultrasound are useful in distinguishing an upper tract tumor from other radiolucent filling defects, such as a uric acid stone. When doubt remains, ureteroscopy with or without biopsy can establish the diagnosis with a high degree of accuracy. Once the diagnosis of upper tract TCC is established, a chest radiograph and liver function tests are needed to evaluate for metastases. A bone scan is indicated for patients with elevated alkaline phosphatase, pain, or other clinical manifestations of disease.

The staging of renal pelvic TCC, outlined below, is similar to that of bladder TCC. The stage and grade correlate closely with survival.

Staging of Transitional Cell Carcinoma of the Renal Pelvis

	Grabstald System	TNM System
Confined to mucosa	O	TaTis
Invasion of lamina propria	A	T1
Invasion of muscularis	B	T2
Extension into fat or renal parenchyma	C	T3
Spread to adjacent organs	D	T4
Lymph node spread	D	N+
Distant metastases	D	M+

Total nephroureterectomy, including a cuff of bladder, is the treatment of choice in patients with localized, unilateral, renal pelvic TCC and a normal, functioning contralateral kidney. The 5-year survival rate following nephroureterectomy for patients with low-grade, noninvasive renal pelvic TCC is 75–90%. A conservative approach is indicated in patients with a solitary kidney, bilateral disease, or with marginal renal function. Surgical options include a partial nephrectomy, open pyelotomy with tumor excision, or endoscopic excision either percutaneously or ureteroscopically. Recurrences are common, and patients must be followed meticulously. Topical immunotherapy using bacille Calmette-Guérin (BCG) and chemotherapy have been reported successful.

In the present patient, intravenous urography, retrograde pyelography (note filling defect in figure), and cytologic study confirmed the diagnosis of urothelial cancer. A right nephroureterectomy was performed, and pathology showed grade II/III TCC confined to the renal pelvis, with invasion into the muscularis. She is receiving BCG and chemotherapy and is being followed closely.

Clinical Pearls

1. Transitional cell carcinoma of the renal pelvis features bilateral involvement in 2–5% of patients.
2. Approximately 30–50% of patients with renal pelvic TCC subsequently develop TCC of the bladder.
3. Approximately 2–4% of patients with bladder cancer have upper tract TCC.

REFERENCES

1. Grabstald H, Whitmore WF, Melamed MR: Renal pelvic tumors. JAMA 218:845–854, 1971.
2. Hudson MA, Catalona WJ: Urothelial tumors of the bladder, upper tracts, and prostate. In Gillenwater JY, Grayhack JT, Howards SS, Duckett JW (eds): Adult and Pediatric Urology, 3rd ed. St. Louis, Mosby, 1996.

PATIENT 28

A 71-year-old woman with dysuria, hematuria, and low back pain

A 71-year-old woman presents with dysuria, frequent urination, intermittent gross hematuria, and chronic low back pain. She has a history of three urinary tract infections in the past 12 months, including one episode of acute pyelonephritis. Each infection was empirically treated with oral antibiotics, with resolution of symptoms. The patient has no previous urologic history.

Physical Examination: Vital signs: normal. Abdomen: soft; mild, bilateral costovertebral angle tenderness. Genitalia: normal. Rectal: normal.

Laboratory Findings: BUN 20 mg/dl, creatinine 1.5 mg/dl. WBC 14,400/μl, with normal differential. Urinalysis: pH 8.0, leukocyte esterase 3+, nitrite positive, WBC > 25/hpf, RBC > 25/hpf, large bacteria. Urine culture: > 100,000 colony-forming units of *Proteus mirabilis*. Abdominal radiograph: see figure.

Question: Describe the relationship between the patient's clinical problem and the radiographic findings.

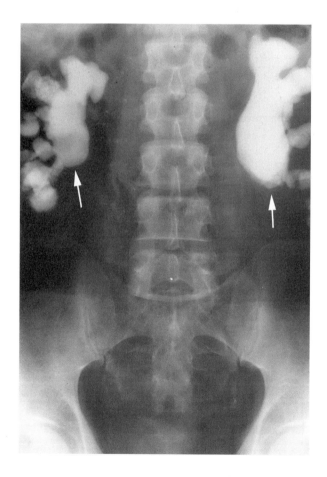

Diagnosis: Recurrent urinary tract infection with *Proteus mirabilis* and bilateral staghorn calculi

Discussion: The finding of recurrent urinary tract infection with the organism *Proteus mirabilis* should raise the suspicion of a persistent upper urinary tract source—specifically, an infection stone. *P. mirabilis* is a urea-splitting bacteria that produces the enzyme urease. Urea is converted to ammonia and carbon dioxide, which results in an alkaline urine and leads to supersaturation of magnesium ammonium phosphate and carbonate apatite and formation of struvite stones. The formation of these struvite stones in the renal collecting system leads to the staghorn configuration typically seen with this type of stone.

It is unknown whether the initiating factor is the stone or the infection. Infection with the typical pathogens is required to establish the conditions in which struvite stone formation can occur. On the other hand, the presence of a stone can serve as a nidus for infection with these organisms and certainly can make it more difficult to eradicate the infection with conventional antibiotic therapy. In addition to *P. mirabilis*, other common urease-producing bacteria include *Klebsiella, Serratia, Pseudomonas*, and *Staphylococcus. Escherichia coli* does not produce urease.

Urinary tract infections caused by urease-producing organisms should prompt evaluation of the upper urinary tracts, especially in recurrent infections. Plain abdominal radiography reveals the presence of most stones. Intravenous urography allows examination of the anatomy of the collecting system and a functional assessment of the kidneys. Metabolic evaluation also is important, since an undiagnosed metabolic problem could predispose to recurrent stone formation despite adequate primary treatment. Metabolic disease can be a factor in the pathogenesis of up to 30% of staghorn calculi.

Treatment consists of eradicating infection and achieving a stone-free state. Conservative therapy or observation is associated with a significant mortality rate of up to 28% and places the patient at risk of additional life-threatening renal infections. Therefore, aggressive treatment of the stone disease is warranted. The management of staghorn calculi has evolved dramatically over the past 20 years. Prior to the development of minimally invasive stone therapy, open surgery with pyelolithotomy, anatrophic nephrolithotomy, and nephrectomy were the only methods available to eradicate the stone. Since the development of extra-corporeal shock wave lithotripsy (ESWL) and percutaneous nephrolithotomy, most staghorn calculi now can be eradicated successfully with one or a combination of these minimally invasive techniques. The key to successful treatment remains removal of the stone burden in its entirety and prevention of stone recurrence. Antibiotic therapy before, during, and after surgery also is critical to achieving success and preventing septic complications.

In the present patient, abdominal radiography demonstrated stones in the upper urinary tract (see figure, *arrows*). ESWL and percutaneous nephrolithotomy were performed, with successful eradication. She completed a course of ampicillin and gentamicin (begun preoperatively) and has had no further complications.

Clinical Pearls

1. Recurrent urinary tract infection with urease-producing organisms should raise suspicion of infection stones.

2. Infection or struvite stones are composed of magnesium ammonium phosphate and carbonate apatite, which precipitate in an alkaline urine infected with urease-producing organisms.

3. In most cases, aggressive treatment of staghorn calculi is indicated to prevent potential life-threatening infections and progressive renal deterioration.

REFERENCES
1. Blandy JP, Singh M: The case for a more aggressive approach to staghorn stones. J Urol 115:505–506, 1976.
2. Spirnak JP, Resnick MI: Urinary stones. In Tanagho EA, McAninch JW (eds): Smith's General Urology, 13th ed. Norwalk, CT, Appleton & Lange, 1992.
3. Wang LP, Wong HY, Griffith DP: Treatment options in struvite stones. Urol Clin North Am 24(1):149–162, 1997.

PATIENT 29

A 51-year-old man with bilateral hydronephrosis and azotemia

A 51-year-old man presents with a 6-month history of progressively worsening obstructive voiding symptoms including hesitancy, intermittency, weak force of stream, and sensation of incomplete bladder emptying. He also reports frequent urination during the day and night, voiding every 1–2 hours. However, he has been unable to initiate voiding for 4–5 days prior to presentation, except for frequent but minimal dribbling. The patient complains of lower abdominal pain, radiating to the back; lethargy; fatigue; nausea; and vomiting of 1-week duration.

Physical Examination: Vital signs: normal. Abdomen: soft; moderate infraumbilical tenderness; suprapubic distension to umbilicus. Genitalia: uncircumcised phallus with urinary dribbling; normal testes. Rectal: symmetrical 30- to 40-gram prostate; no nodules.

Laboratory Findings: BUN 59 mg/dl, creatinine 5.1 mg/dl, potassium 5.4 mEq/L. Prostatic specific antigen: 3.5 ng/ml. Urinalysis: pH 5.5, WBC 3–5/hpf, RBC 3–5/hpf. Abdominal radiograph: normal. Renal ultrasound: see figure.

Question: The patient's symptoms and azotemia began to resolve within hours of Foley catheterization. What is the most likely etiology of this patient's hydronephrosis and renal failure?

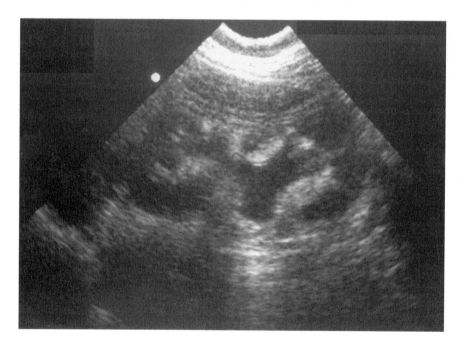

Diagnosis: Urinary retention and complete bladder outlet obstruction, most likely from benign prostatic hyperplasia

Discussion: The progressively worsening obstructive voiding symptoms in this patient, eventually leading to what appeared to be urinary retention with overflow dribbling or incontinence, is highly suggestive of bladder outlet obstruction secondary to prostatic enlargement. Associated symptoms of nausea, vomiting, fatigue, and lethargy can be attributed to the patient's azotemia.

The lower abdominal distension should be interpreted as a distended bladder, until proven otherwise. The enlarged prostate on rectal examination suggests, but does not guarantee, prostatic obstruction. Gland enlargement does not predict the degree of obstruction; acute renal failure is defined by the elevated BUN and creatinine. The clinical picture in this patient suggests a postrenal or obstructive etiology for renal failure. Level of obstruction is determined by the clinical findings. Bladder catheterization revealing a large urinary residual volume is consistent with bladder outlet obstruction. A renal and bladder ultrasound also can determine the level of obstruction. The presence of a relatively empty bladder (prior to catheter placement) with bilateral hydroureteronephrosis indicates obstruction in the distal ureters or ureterovesical junctions. The presence of bilateral hydronephrosis with nondilated ureters suggests a more proximal ureteric obstruction, possibly secondary to extrinsic compression.

Based on the clinical findings, this patient suffered acute renal failure secondary to urinary retention from bladder outlet obstruction. The renal failure was reversible following bladder decompression. After relief of acute obstruction, it is necessary to watch carefully for a postobstructive diuresis. Urinary output and electrolytes should be monitored closely. Adequate intravenous or oral hydration is required until renal urinary concentrating ability returns to baseline. Electrolyte imbalances should be corrected.

After the initial management, treatment of this condition can take multiple pathways. An episode of acute urinary retention generally implies end-stage bladder decompensation in the face of progressively worsening outlet obstruction. Spontaneous voiding after catheter removal is unlikely in these patients. Exceptions include urinary retention secondary to medications (alpha-agonists or anticholinergics), infection (acute bacterial prostatitis), and postoperative urinary retention. If any of these factors are present, there is a reasonably good chance the patient will regain spontaneous voiding after the removal of the inciting factor and a period of continuous bladder decompression.

Except for those who are poor surgical candidates, patients suffering acute urinary retention secondary to benign prostatic hyperplasia (BPH) should be considered for surgical treatment. Nonsurgical treatment for refractory urinary retention includes chronic indwelling catheter (urethral or suprapubic) or clean intermittent catheterization. These therapies are not ideal and increase the risk of infectious complications. Refractory urinary retention, recurrent urinary tract infections secondary to BPH, recurrent or persistent gross hematuria from BPH, concomitant bladder stones, and renal insufficiency due to chronic bladder outlet obstruction are all accepted indications for surgical intervention.

The most common surgical treatment is transurethral resection of the prostate (TURP). In certain cases featuring unusually large prostate glands, large bladder calculi, a large bladder diverticulum, or a significant intravesical gland component, open prostatectomy (via a suprapubic or retropubic approach) may be indicated or preferred. Recent advances in minimally-invasive endoscopic treatments include balloon dilation therapy, intraprostatic stents, electrovaporization, microwave therapy, laser prostatectomy, and the use of radio frequency energy. Many of these modalities are still undergoing investigation, and their ultimate role in the surgical treatment of BPH has yet to be completely defined.

In the present patient, the diagnosis of bladder outlet obstruction causing acute renal failure was confirmed by the relief of obstruction following urethral catheterization and subsequent resolution of the acute renal failure. The patient did experience a mild, self-limited post-obstructive diuresis, and the BUN and creatinine returned to normal levels. Hydroureteronephrosis also resolved on repeat renal ultrasonography. Following resolution of the renal failure, the patient was treated with transurethral prostatectomy. Pathologic examination of prostatic tissue revealed benign glandular hyperplasia. The patient had significantly improved voiding function following surgery, without evidence of residual obstruction.

Clinical Pearls

1. Immediate bladder drainage with catheterization is the initial management of acute urinary retention and azotemia resulting from bladder outlet obstruction.

2. A postobstructive diuresis can ensue following bladder decompression. Urinary output and electrolyte monitoring should be instituted. Volume and electrolyte replacement may be necessary.

3. Refractory urinary retention secondary to BPH is one of the accepted indications for surgical treatment of BPH.

REFERENCES

1. McConnell JD, Barry MS, Bruskewitz RC, et al: Benign Prostatic Hyperplasia: Diagnosis and Treatment. Clinical Practice Guideline No. 8. Publication No. 94-0582. Rockville, MD, U.S. Department of Health and Human Services, Agency for Health Care Policy and Research, 1994.
2. Grayhack JT, Kozlowski JM: Benign prostatic hyperplasia. In Gillenwater JY, Grayhack JT, Howards SS, Duckett JW (eds): Adult and Pediatric Urology, 3rd ed. St. Louis, Mosby, 1996.

PATIENT 30

A 28-year-old man with acute flank pain

A 28-year-old man complains of an acute onset of right flank pain, with periodic increases in intensity. He also experienced chills, nausea, and vomiting soon after the onset of pain. The patient denies voiding problems and hematuria. He has been working as an outdoor construction worker during the summer months and is otherwise healthy.

Physical Examination: Temperature 38.4; pulse 88; respirations 16; blood pressure 154/70. Abdomen: soft; moderate right-sided tenderness with right costovertebral angle tenderness; no peritoneal signs. Genitourinary: normal. Rectal: normal.

Laboratory Findings: Electrolytes, BUN, and creatinine: normal. WBC 16,000/μl with left shift. Urinalysis: pH 5.0, leukocyte esterase positive, nitrite negative, 5–10 WBC/hpf, > 25 RBC/hpf. Abdominal radiograph: normal. Noncontrast spiral computed tomography (CT) scan of abdomen and pelvis: see figure.

Question: What is the etiology of this patient's acute flank pain?

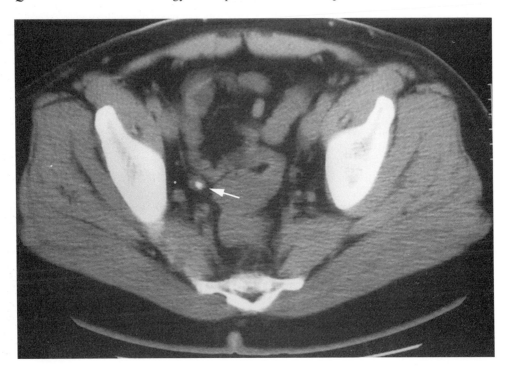

Diagnosis: Obstructing right ureteral, uric acid calculus

Discussion: This patient's pain and the associated symptoms of nausea and vomiting are consistent with renal colic. The presence of microscopic hematuria also is expected with urolithiasis. These findings alone should raise the suspicion for an obstructing urinary tract stone. The plain abdominal radiograph revealed no pathologic calcifications. However, only about 90% of urinary stones are radiopaque. Pure uric acid stones are radiolucent and will not be demonstrated on a plain abdominal x-ray. Other imaging studies are required to make the diagnosis.

Intravenous urography has been the traditional imaging study to evaluate flank pain and suspected obstructing calculus. An intravenous urogram, not performed in this patient, may have demonstrated delay of contrast excretion with or without a characteristic filling defect secondary to a radiolucent uric acid stone. **Noncontrast CT scans** are an excellent modality for demonstrating uric acid lithiasis. All urinary stones have a high attenuation appearance on CT scan; uric acid stones have attenuation values in the 300–400 range.

At many institutions, noncontrast helical CT scan is replacing intravenous urography as the initial imaging modality to evaluate flank pain. It offers distinct advantages in terms of speed, avoidance of both oral and intravenous contrast, more precise anatomic localization of the stone, and the potential for locating other abdominal or pelvic etiologies for pain outside the urinary tract. CT scan and intravenous urography have been shown to be of equal value in determining the presence or absence of obstruction, but CT performs better in identifying the actual stone.

The urinary pH also is critical in making the diagnosis of uric acid stone. Uric acid is the major endproduct of purine metabolism. The formation of uric acid stones is related to the urinary supersaturation of undissociated uric acid. Urine pH and uric acid concentration are the prime factors determining supersaturation. At urine pH below 5.5, most of the uric acid remains in the insoluble, undissociated form, leading to crystallization and stone formation. Uric acid concentration is dependent upon urinary volume and uric acid excretion. Chronic dehydration states can lead to low urinary volumes, while increased uric acid excretion can be caused by increased endogenous production or diets rich in purine-containing foods (e.g., meats, poultry, fish).

Uric acid calculi, unlike other, more common stone types, can be successfully treated with medical therapy. Treatment is aimed at elevating the urine pH and decreasing uric acid concentration by increasing urine volume and decreasing uric acid excretion. Urine alkalinization to achieve 6.5–7.0 urinary pH can be accomplished with oral agents such as potassium citrate or sodium bicarbonate, or with intravenous 1/6 molar lactate infusion. A total daily urinary output of 2 liters is desirable. Uric acid excretion can be decreased by diets low in purine-rich foods and the use of allopurinol, a xanthine oxidase inhibitor.

Occasionally, surgical intervention is required. High-grade obstruction, intractable renal colic, coexisting infection, and renal insufficiency are all indications for surgical intervention in the form of urinary drainage procedures.

In the present patient, a CT scan demonstrated a high-attenuation structure in the distal right ureter (see figure, *arrow*), which is the ureteral calculus. There also was an increase of the renal cortical thickness in the ipsilateral kidney, a secondary sign of obstruction. He had associated infection, manifested by fever, leukocytosis, and pyuria. Thus, retrograde ureteral stent placement was required to decompress the obstructed kidney. The symptoms resolved, at which time the stone was treated with medical dissolution therapy.

Clinical Pearls

1. Uric acid calculi represent 5–10% of all urinary stones in the United States.
2. Urine pH < 5.5 predisposes to uric acid stone formation.
3. Pure uric acid stones are radiolucent on plain abdominal radiographs, but noncontrast CT scan reveals uric acid stones with attenuation values in the 300–400 range.
4. Uric acid stones are highly amenable to medical therapy, generally aimed at elevating urinary pH into the 6.5–7.0 range and optimizing urinary volume to more than 2 liters per day.

REFERENCES
1. Resnick MI: Uric acid stones. In Resnick MI, Kursh ED (eds): Current Therapy in Genitourinary Surgery, 2nd ed. St. Louis, Mosby, 1992.
2. Spirnak JP, Resnick MI: Urinary stones. In Tanagho EA, McAninch JW (eds): Smith's General Urology, 13th ed. Norwalk, CT, Appleton & Lange, 1992.
3. Koelliker SL, Cronan JJ: Acute urinary tract obstruction: Imaging update. Urol Clin North Am 24(3):571–582, 1997.
4. Low RK, Stoller ML: Uric acid-related nephrolithiasis. Urol Clin North Am 24(1):135–148, 1997.

PATIENT 31

A 26-year-old man with infertility and a scrotal mass

A 26-year-old married man presents with a 15-month history of inability to conceive. He is otherwise healthy, and there is no history of endocrinologic or urologic disorders. He has never fathered a child. The patient has been married for 2 years to a 26-year-old woman who also is healthy and has never been pregnant. His wife has undergone a complete gynecologic workup for female infertility, which was negative.

Physical Examination: General: normal appearance. Genitalia: circumcised phallus without abnormalities; testis bilaterally palpable, with area along left spermatic cord that feels like "a bunch of worms"; right testicle appears normal until patient performs Valsalva maneuver—then structural cluster similar to that along left spermatic cord is noted.

Laboratory Findings: Serum testosterone, follicle-stimulating hormone, luteinizing hormone levels: normal. Semen analysis: volume 2.4 ml (normal 1.5–5 ml), sperm density 12 million cells/ml (normal > 20 million), motility 20% (normal > 50%), morphology (measured by strict criteria of Kruger) 15% (normal > 14%).

Question: What is your diagnosis?

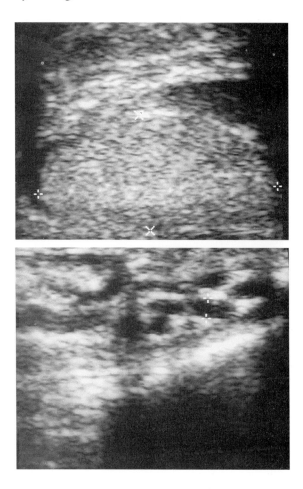

Diagnosis: Bilateral varicocele

Discussion: Male-factor infertility is responsible for failure to conceive in approximately 20–30% of infertile couples. Scrotal varices, or varicoceles, represent the most common reversible cause, although 15% of *all* men have some degree of varicocele, and the majority of these do not have difficulty conceiving. Nonetheless, varicoceles have been observed in 19–41% of all men being treated for infertility, and may be seen in as many as 60% of men presenting with secondary infertility (i.e., failure to conceive after prior successful attempts).

The mechanism of spermatogenic injury from varicoceles is unclear. Some studies suggest that varicoceles result in elevated testicular temperatures unfavorable to spermatogenesis. Others suggest subtle hormonal changes from progressive damage to the testicle. It also has been hypothesized that there may be reflux of toxic metabolites from the renal or adrenal vein into the gonadal venous system, especially on the left, where varicoceles are more common and the gonadal vein comes directly off of the renal vein.

The Valsalva maneuver always should be performed in the infertile male patient during standing examination to elicit the presence of varicocele. The serpiginous nature of the dilated veins of the varicocele is evident on touch, and the varicocele typically is described as feeling like "a bunch of worms." Some varicoceles are only detectable by color-flow Doppler ultrasound, however, and are referred to as subclinical. Their significance in male-factor infertility is controversial.

Ultrasound of a patient's scrotum using a 7.5 megahertz transducer reveals a homogenous internal texture of the normal testicle (see *top* figure; crosses outline the testicle). During the Valsalva maneuver, a dilated vein, or varicocele, is evident in the spermatic cord (*bottom* figure; crosses).

Repair of varicoceles is a relatively simple, outpatient procedure. Varicocelectomy involves tying off all visible venous structures while preserving the arterial and lymphatic supply. Many surgeons today prefer to perform the operation under magnification, either employing operating loupes or a microscope. The approach may be retroperitoneal, inguinal, or subinguinal. Sperm density, morphology, and motility may all improve after varicocelectomy; sperm motility reportedly is most affected. Most importantly, pregnancy rates after varicocele repair approach 50%.

The present patient had a bilateral lesion, the right side of which was observable only during the Valsalva maneuver. Ultrasound was unnecessary, however, as the lesion was detectable by physical examination. He elected to undergo a bilateral varicocelectomy. The operation was performed without incident under local anesthesia with intravenous sedation. Three months later, a semen analysis showed normalization of the sperm density and motility, and the couple conceived their first child shortly thereafter.

Clinical Pearls

1. Varicoceles represent an important cause of reversible male-factor infertility and must be carefully screened for by physical examination.
2. Surgical correction of varicoceles results in a high rate of successful pregnancies.

REFERENCES
1. Schlesinger MH, Wilets IF, Nagler HM: Treatment outcome after varicocelectomy: A critical analysis. Urol Clin North Am 21(3):517–529, 1994.
2. Thompson ST: Prevention of male infertility: An update. Urol Clin North Am 21(3):365–376, 1994.
3. Junnila J, Lassen P: Testicular masses. Am Fam Phys 57(4):685–692, 1998.

PATIENT 32

A 72-year-old man with abdominal pain and a large flank mass

A 72-year-old man with a history of vague abdominal discomfort and normal esophagogastro-duodenoscopy (EGD) presents with the acute onset of abdominal pain. The patient denies symptoms of nausea, vomiting, and fever, change in bowel habits, and hematuria. He also denies prior surgery or current use of medications.

Physical Examination: Temperature 37.2°; pulse 110; respirations 12; blood pressure 90/55. General: well-nourished; obvious discomfort. Lymph nodes: no lymphadenopathy. Chest: clear. Cardiac: tachycardic with strong pulses and no murmur. Abdomen: soft; left-sided diffuse tenderness in absence of peritoneal signs. Back: large (8 × 8 cm) left flank mass tender to palpation. Genitalia: normal. Digital rectal exam: normal prostate, no mass.

Laboratory Findings: Electrolytes, BUN, creatinine: normal. WBC normal, hemoglobin 8.5 g/dl, Hct 26%. Stool: guaiac negative. Urinalysis and urine culture: negative. Urgent computerized tomography (CT) scan of abdomen: see figure.

Question: What is the diagnosis, based on the presentation and CT scan findings?

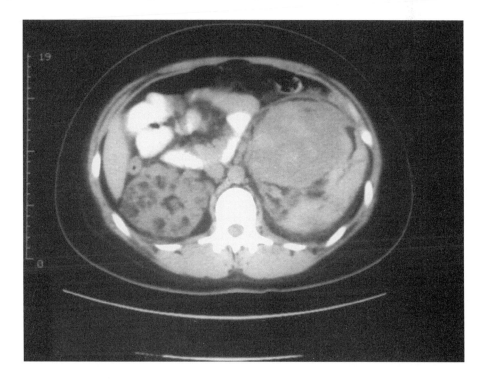

Diagnosis: Bilateral renal angiomyolipomas with left-sided rupture and retroperitoneal hemorrhage

Discussion: Renal angiomyolipoma (AML) is a benign, solid tumor characterized by the presence of variable elements of fat, blood vessels, and muscle cells. Renal AMLs commonly are bilateral and have a proclivity for multiplicity, hemorrhage, and large size. There is a definitive association between tuberous sclerosis and AML, as roughly 80% of patients with tuberous sclerosis have AMLs. In these patients, the tumors typically are bilateral yet asymptomatic. In patients without associated tuberous sclerosis, AML most commonly is unilateral and may present with abdominal or flank pain, mass, hematuria, or retroperitoneal hemorrhage. AML also may present with gastrointestinal symptoms related to mass effect or as an incidental finding on cross-sectional imaging performed for other reasons.

Ultrasonographic characteristics of AML include a sharply marginated, uniform mass with markedly increased echogenicity usually equivalent to the renal sinus. Interestingly, increased serendipitous discovery of small renal masses by ultrasound has coincided with increased detection of small hyperechoic renal cell carcinomas that mimic AML. Ultrasound differentiation of AML from hyperechoic renal cell carcinoma is problematic, but the presence of acoustic shadowing suggests AML, whereas a hypoechoic rim or the presence of intratumoral cystic lesions is suspicious for renal cell carcinoma. Recent reports suggest that special techniques such as measurement of ultrasonic frequency-dependent attenuation may help in distinction of AML from renal cell carcinoma. Nonetheless, CT or MRI presently must be done for further characterization of hyperechoic masses found on ultrasound. Once a confident diagnosis of AML is rendered, ultrasound also is reliable in the clinical followup of asymptomatic small lesions, as only AMLs larger than 4 centimeters are particularly prone to hemorrhage.

Vascular and muscular elements give AML a variegated appearance on CT, but the presence of fat density (-20 to -80 Hounsfield units) virtually is diagnostic. Disturbingly, the recent literature describes cases of renal cell carcinoma with admixtures of fat density on CT. However, every case of renal cell carcinoma with fatty elements also reveals concomitant calcifications, which are not present with AML. Therefore, fat density on CT in the absence of calcifications invariably excludes renal cell carcinoma from diagnosis. Novel advances in CT imaging techniques show further promise in detection of fat in renal lesions as small as 0.4 centimeters.

The role of MRI in the evaluation of AML is still evolving. Fat suppression techniques are especially helpful in the diagnosis of AML by MRI because high signal intensity of AML on T-1 and T-2 weighted images is nonspecific, whereas low signal intensity with fat saturation images confirms the presence of fatty elements. Further refinements in MRI, such as chemical shift and in-phase/out-of-phase fat suppression sequences, hold great potential in the differentiation of even small AMLs from renal cell carcinoma.

The management of AML is somewhat controversial but depends upon symptoms, tumor size, and the accuracy of preoperative diagnosis. Tumors less than 4 centimeters rarely cause symptoms; these patients may be followed conservatively with serial imaging via ultrasound or CT. Unfortunately, roughly one-half of these small tumors will progress in size, necessitating more aggressive treatment. Asymptomatic tumors larger than 4.0 centimeters as well as symptomatic AMLs should be treated with attempted nephron-sparing modalities, such as angioinfarction or partial nephrectomy, due to frequent multiplicity and bilaterality. Renal cell carcinoma can coexist in patients with AML (although rarely); thus, tumors should be excised if they contain calcifications or lack any of the radiographic characteristics of AML. Renal AML usually follows a benign course without metastases, but aggressive local behavior is well-documented, with reports of extrarenal extension, hilar lymph node involvement, and invasion of the renal vein or inferior vena cava with tumor thrombus. Venous or lymphatic involvement represents only local invasion, as pathologic examination invariably lacks malignant transformation.

The present patient was aggressively resuscitated with IV fluids and transfused to a hemoglobin of 10 g/dl. He underwent successful angioinfarction in the acute setting to stop active bleeding. After convalescence from the acute retroperitoneal hemorrhage, he subsequently had a partial nephrectomy secondary to continued abdominal pain from mass effect.

Clinical Pearls

1. Angiomyolipomas are composed of an admixture of abnormal blood vessels, smooth muscle cells, and fatty elements, but one cell type may predominate.

2. The majority of AMLs are *not* associated with tuberous sclerosis. However, roughly 80% of patients *with* tuberous sclerosis will eventually manifest AMLs.

3. Tuberous sclerosis is an autosomal dominant condition characterized by the triad of epilepsy, mental retardation, and adenoma sebaceum; hamartomas of the kidneys, brain, eye, bones, heart, and lungs also are characteristic.

4. As a general rule of thumb, AMLs smaller than 4.0 centimeters may be managed expectantly with serial imaging; those larger than 4.0 centimeters or symptomatic tumors should be treated with nephron-sparing surgery or embolization.

5. Fat density on CT virtually is diagnostic of AML, and in the absence of calcifications essentially excludes renal cell carcinoma from consideration.

REFERENCES

1. Forman HP, Middleton WD, Melson GL, et al: Hyperechoic renal cell carcinomas: Increase in detection at US. Radiology 188:431–434, 1993.
2. Hobarth K, Klingler C, Kuber W, et al: Value of routine sonography in the diagnosis and conservative management of renal angiomyolipoma. European Urol 24:239–243, 1993.
3. Baert J, Vandamme B, Sciot R, et al: Benign angiomyolipoma involving the renal vein and vena cava as a tumor thrombus: Case report. J Urol 153:1205–1207, 1995.
4. Leder RA: Genitourinary case of the day. Am J Roentgenol 165:198–199, 1995.
5. Lemaitre L, Robert Y, Dubrulle F, et al: Renal angiomyolipoma: Growth followed up with CT and/or US. Radiology 197:598–602, 1995.
6. Rodriguez R, Fishman EK, Marshall FF: Differential diagnosis and evaluation of the incidentally discovered renal mass. Semin Urol Oncol 13:246–253, 1995.
7. Cittadini G Jr, Mucelli FP, Danza FM, et al: "Aggressive" renal angiomyolipoma. Acta Radiologica 37:927–932, 1996.
8. Jennings SB, Linehan WM: Renal, perirenal, and ureteral neoplasms. In Gillenwater JY, Grayhack JT, Howards SS, et al (eds): Adult and Pediatric Urology. St. Louis, MO, Mosby Year-Book, Inc., 1996, pp 643–694.
9. Siegel CL, Middleton WD, Teefey SA, et al: Angiomyolipoma and renal cell carcinoma: US differentiation. Radiology 198:789–793, 1996.
10. Henderson RJ, Germany R, Peavy PW, et al: Fat density in renal cell carcinoma: Demonstration with computerized tomography. J Urol 157:1347–1348, 1997.
11. Taniguchi N, Itoh K, Nakamura S, et al: Differentiation of renal cell carcinomas from angiomyolipomas by ultrasonic frequency dependent attenuation. J Urol 157:1242–1245, 1997.

PATIENT 33

A 72-year-old man with a cystic mass of the kidney

A 72-year-old man with a history of hypertension and coronary artery disease status post coronary artery bypass grafting (CABG) was thought to have a questionable pulsatile abdominal mass by his internist. The internist obtained a computed tomography scan of the abdomen to rule out abdominal aortic aneurysm, and an incidental left renal mass was discovered. The patient denies chest pain, shortness of breath, exertional dyspnea, claudication, abdominal pain, and urinary symptoms. Medications include a beta-blocker and an angiotensin-converting enzyme (ACE) inhibitor.

Physical Examination: Normal.

Laboratory Findings: CBC, electrolytes, BUN, creatinine: normal. Liver function tests: normal. Urinalysis: normal. Urine culture: negative. Computed tomography (CT) scan of abdomen (see figure): lesion did not enhance after administration of intravenous contrast.

Question: What is the Bosniak category of the left renal cystic mass?

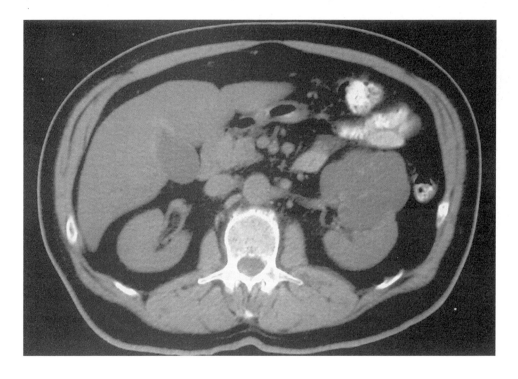

Diagnosis: Bosniak category 2 or minimally complicated renal cyst

Discussion: The vast majority of renal cysts are incidentally discovered upon abdominal imaging for an unrelated process. Simple cysts are the most common renal masses. They must be readily differentiated from complex cystic lesions and solid masses by radiographic means to avoid unnecessary procedures. Lesions with sharply marginated, almost imperceptible walls; lack of internal echoes; and good through transmission with acoustic enhancement of the posterior wall meet strict sonographic criteria for simple cysts and do not require further evaluation. Complex cysts are characterized sonographically by variability in shape, indistinct borders, the presence of septae or calcifications, varying degrees of internal echoes, and even solid or nodular components. Complex cystic or solid lesions on ultrasound mandate further evaluation with CT.

The Bosniak classification categorizes cystic lesions based on key CT findings in an attempt to accurately delineate malignant risk. Bosniak category 1 includes **simple benign** cysts, with CT characteristics including uniform water density with low attenuation (0–20 Hounsfield units [H.U.]), sharply marginated borders with smooth walls, and the absence of contrast enhancement. These criteria virtually exclude malignancy, and no further workup is necessary.

Bosniak category 2 lesions or **minimally complicated** cysts contain thin, nonenhancing septae or linear, minimal calcifications. Category 2 also includes the hyperdense renal cyst, which by strict definition is a small (less than 3 centimeters), nonenhancing mass with sharply marginated, smooth walls that is homogeneously hyperdense (40–49 H.U.) on precontrast CT. The vast majority of all class 2 lesions are benign, with rare exceptions. This led to development of Bosniak category 2F, or minimally complex cysts that require followup imaging due to radiographic suspicion of malignancy. Unfortunately, criteria for differentiation between class 2 and 2F lesions are not well defined. Ultimately, Bosniak category 2 lesions have very low malignant risk and may be followed conservatively.

Bosniak category 3 includes equivocal lesions or **moderately complicated** cysts, with thickened, complex septae or dense, irregular calcifications. The malignant risk of these lesions is intermediate; roughly 50% of Bosniak category 3 lesions ultimately prove to be malignant. Class 3 lesions warrant surgical exploration or biopsy with either radical or partial nephrectomy, as indicated, due to uncertain malignant potential.

Bosniak category 4 or **cystic malignancy** includes cystic masses with solid or nodular components; irregular, thick margins; or the presence of unequivocal contrast-enhancement. These lesions should be considered renal cell carcinomas until proven otherwise and extirpated with either partial or radical nephrectomy.

The present patient met strict criteria for a minimally complicated cyst with subsequent negligible risk of malignancy. His category 2 Bosniak lesion was managed conservatively with observation.

Clinical Pearls

1. The majority of renal masses identified on intravenous urography are simple cysts, for which ultrasound is very accurate in diagnosis.

2. Autopsy studies estimate that approximately 50% of the population over 50 years of age have grossly evident renal parenchymal cysts.

3. Unequivocal contrast enhancement is defined as an increase in density of at least 20 H.U. after intravenous administration of contrast.

4. Von-Hippel-Lindau disease and tuberous sclerosis are both autosomal dominant disorders which may manifest with multiple, bilateral renal cysts.

5. Simple renal cysts are rare in children and unreported in neonates.

REFERENCES
1. Coleman BG: Ultrasonography of the upper genitourinary tract. Urol Clin North Am 12:633–644, 1985.
2. Bosniak MA: The current radiological approach to renal cysts. Radiology 158:1–10, 1986.
3. Aronson S, Frazier HA, Baluch JD, et al: Cystic renal masses: Usefulness of the Bosniak classification. Urol Radiol 13:83–90, 1991.
4. Bosniak MA: Difficulties in classifying cystic lesions of the kidney. Urol Radiol 13:91–93, 1991.
5. Bosniak MA: Problems in the radiologic diagnosis of renal parenchymal tumors. Urol Clin North Am 20:217–230, 1993.
6. Curry NS, Bissada NK: Radiologic evaluation of small and indeterminant renal masses. Urol Clin North Am 24:493–505, 1997.
7. Haas CA, Resnick MI: Office-based ultrasound for urologists. AUA Update Series 16:242–247, 1997.

PATIENT 34

A 69-year-old man with a solid renal mass

A 69-year-old otherwise healthy man presents with a 3-day history of gross, painless, total hematuria. The patient denies any prior medical or urologic history. He has not experienced weight loss or other constitutional symptoms and has never smoked.

Physical Examination: Vital signs: normal. General: healthy looking, appears comfortable. Lymph nodes: no lymphadenopathy. Chest: clear. Abdomen: soft, no mass. Back: no flank tenderness or mass. Genitalia: normal. Digital rectal exam: normal.

Laboratory Findings: Hct 28%, WBC and electrolytes normal, hemoglobin 9 g/dl. Liver function tests: normal. Calcium and BUN normal; creatinine 1 mg/dl. Urinalysis: RBC too numerous to count. Urine culture: negative. Intravenous urogram: suspicious for left renal mass. Office flexible cystoscopy: normal. Computed tomography (CT) scan of abdomen: see figure.

Question: What is the most probable *specific* pathologic diagnosis based on the presentation and CT findings?

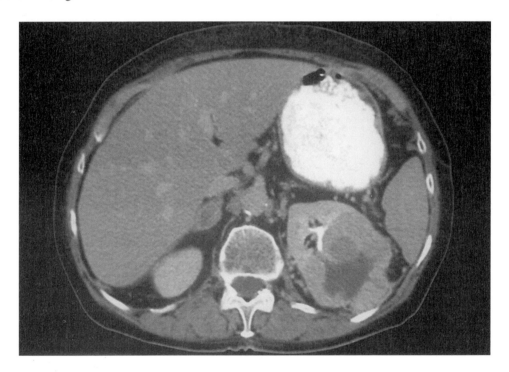

Diagnosis: Clear cell renal cell carcinoma

Discussion: Renal cell carcinoma (RCC) accounts for roughly 90% of all primary malignant renal tumors and is estimated to account for about 28,000 new cancer diagnoses and over 11,000 deaths in the United States alone. Symptoms are myriad and include the "too-late triad" of abdominal pain, mass, and hematuria. This triad rarely is present and typically is a harbinger of advanced disease. In the current era of ubiquitous cross-sectional imaging, incidental discovery with ultrasound or CT has become the most common presentation of a renal mass.

Intravenous urogram often is the initial diagnostic study, as many patients with RCC present with hematuria. Findings on intravenous urogram suspicious for RCC include mass effect, abnormalities in renal contour, and distortion or displacement of the collecting system. Nephrotomography improves visualization of the collecting system and renal parenchyma by excluding structures not in the desired imaging plane. Despite refinements such as tomography, intravenous urogram still is inferior to other modalities in assessment of renal lesions, especially in detection of small anterior or posterior masses without distortion of renal contour or the collecting system. The implication of mass on intravenous urogram or nephrotomography requires further evaluation with ultrasound or CT.

Diagnosis of RCC is complicated due to the high prevalence of renal lesions, the vast majority of which are benign cysts. The ultrasound characteristics of a solid renal mass include heterogeneous shape with indiscriminate borders, the presence of internal echoes, and acoustic impedance. Unfortunately, ultrasound often cannot distinguish benign solid or complex cystic lesions from RCC, so these lesions discovered on ultrasound mandate further workup with CT. The preoperative diagnosis of RCC sometimes is difficult despite multimodal imaging, due to the varied appearance of benign and malignant lesions. However, CT with and without intravenous contrast is the gold standard for the diagnosis and characterization of renal masses. CT characteristics of RCC are diverse and include: solid mass with contrast-enhancement, speckled or irregular calcifications, asymmetric margins with a thick or nodular wall, hypervascularity, hemorrhage, and necrosis.

CT imaging is important not only in diagnosis of RCC, but also in staging. Overall, CT accuracy for staging varies from 60% to 90% and should include assessment of the renal vein and inferior vena cava, adrenal glands, and regional lymph nodes, as well as evaluation of the liver and lungs for distant metastases. CT findings of RCC venous involvement include filling defects or areas of decreased density, changes of intraluminal vein caliber, and venous enlargement. Regional lymph node metastasis by RCC equates a horrible prognosis, with roughly 10% survival at 5 years. Lymph node metastasis is suggested by enlarged nodes or when several normal-sized nodes are clustered. Lymph nodes greater than 2.0 centimeters in diameter usually contain metastatic disease. However, size criteria for lymph node involvement is problematic because enlargement also may be caused by reactive hyperplasia, and micrometastatic deposits cannot be detected by any current imaging modality. Overall, staging of retroperitoneal lymph node metastases by CT has sensitivity and specificity exceeding 80%.

Improvements in MRI, such as gadolinium, and use of special techniques make MRI increasingly useful in evaluation of renal lesions, particularly smaller masses. Gadolinium was a major impetus for MRI, as the presence of paramagnetic contrast-enhancement is now used to delineate benign versus malignant processes, much like contrast-enhanced CT. Furthermore, gadolinium is less nephrotoxic and thus clinically important in patients with renal insufficiency or previous allergy to iodinated contrast. The most prudent indication for MRI in the evaluation of renal masses is as an adjunct to CT when accurate diagnosis or staging remains in doubt. Compared to CT, advantages of MRI include superior definition of tissue planes and the ability to detect local tumor extension and venous involvement. MRI is particularly good for assessment of the renal vein or inferior vena cava, as it clearly is superior to ultrasound or CT and at least as sensitive as venacavography in the detection of venous tumor thrombi. MRI is likewise valuable in depicting the extent of caval thrombus with regard to the diaphragm, hepatic veins, and right atrium. Overall, staging accuracy of MRI ranges from 80% to 90%, with especially high specificity (97%) for inferior vena cava involvement.

Arteriography plays only a limited role in the evaluation of RCC. It is the most expensive and invasive of all modalities used in the evaluation of renal masses and essentially has been replaced with accurate, noninvasive techniques such as ultrasound, CT, and MRI. Classic findings of RCC on arteriography include hypervascularity, arteriovenous communications, and venous pooling. Currently, the primary use of angiography in patients with RCC is for vascular mapping prior to planned nephron-sparing surgery. Specific indications include RCC in a solitary or horseshoe kidney, bilateral RCC, tumors in patients with von Hippel-Lindau syndrome, and tumor angioinfarction. Angiography also may be beneficial in the evaluation of renal masses in patients with severe hypertension, vascular disease, or other history suggestive of possible coexistent renal artery disease.

Radical nephrectomy remains the gold standard for treatment of clinically localized RCC. Nephron-sparing surgery is gaining widespread acceptance and extended indications, but long-term results are still in evolution. Similarly, use of radical nephrectomy and resection of metastases in the setting of advanced disease either before or after immunotherapy remains controversial.

In the present patient, the CT scan revealed a left renal mass with central necrosis. He had a negative metastatic evaluation and underwent left radical nephrectomy. Final pathology revealed renal cell carcinoma, clear cell type, TNM stage T3aN0M0.

Clinical Pearls

1. Most RCCs originate from epithelial cells of the proximal convoluted tubule.

2. A familial form of RCC characterized by alterations on chromosome 3 is seen in patients with von-Hippel-Lindau syndrome (VHL). The spectrum of VHL includes RCC and renal cysts, pancreatic cysts and tumors, retinal hemangiomas, central nervous system hemangioblastomas, and pheochromocytoma.

3. Hereditary papillary RCC is another familial form of RCC characterized by mutation of the c-met proto-oncogene on chromosome 7.

4. RCC may present with a myriad of paraneoplastic syndromes, the most common of which is anemia. Others include erythrocytosis, hypertension, pyrexia, hypercalcemia, and hepatic dysfunction.

5. Stauffer's syndrome is a paraneoplastic syndrome seen in RCC characterized by nonmetastatic hepatic dysfunction with increased alkaline phosphatase, prolonged prothrombin time, increased a2-globulin, and decreased albumin. Animal studies suggest IL-6 and granulocyte colony–stimulating factor may be etiologic factors.

REFERENCES

1. Newhouse JH: The radiographic evaluation of the patient with renal cancer. Urol Clin N Am 20:231–246, 1993.
2. McClennan BL, Deoye LA: The imaging evaluation of renal cell carcinoma: Diagnosis and staging. Radiol Clin N Am 32:55–69, 1994.
3. Levine E: Renal cell carcinoma: Clinical aspects, imaging diagnosis, and staging. Semin Roentgenol 30:128–148, 1995.
4. Rodriguez R, Fishman EK, Marshall FF: Differential diagnosis and evaluation of the incidentally discovered renal mass. Semin Urol Oncol 13:246–253, 1995.
5. Jennings SB, Linehan WM: Renal, perirenal, and ureteral neoplasms. In Gillenwater JY, Grayhack JT, Howards SS, et al (eds): Adult and Pediatric Urology. St. Louis, MO, Mosby Year-Book, Inc., 1996, pp 643–694.
6. Choyke PL: Detection and staging of renal cancer. Magn Reson Imaging Clin N Am 5:29–47, 1997.
7. Curry NS, Bissada NK: Radiologic evaluation of small and indeterminant renal masses. Urol Clin N Am 24:493–505, 1997.
8. Redman BG, Kawachi M, Schwartz D: Urothelial and kidney cancer. In Pazdur R, Coia LR, Hoskins WJ, et al (eds): Cancer Management: A Multidisciplinary Approach. Medical, Surgical, and Radiation Oncology. Huntington, NY, PRR, 1998, pp 441–448.

PATIENT 35

A 71-year-old man with hyponatremia after a transurethral prostatectomy

After alpha-blockade therapy for benign prostatic hypertrophy failed, a 71-year-old man underwent a transurethral prostatectomy for relief of symptoms. The duration of the procedure was 90 minutes, and it was estimated that 14 liters of glycine irrigation fluid was used. The patient's gland was estimated to be 45 grams. In the recovery room, the patient becomes agitated and confused and complains of blurred vision and nausea.

Physical Examination: Temperature 36.3°; pulse 54; blood pressure 90/50; respirations 24. Oxygen saturation 92% on 4 L nasal canula. General: oriented only to person. Cardiac: bradycardic, no rubs, no murmurs. Chest: bibasilar crackles. Abdomen: benign. Genitalia: 18 French foley catheter with cherry-red urine output.

Laboratory Findings: Hemoglobin 11.4 g/dl (preoperative 12.2). Electrolytes: sodium 120 mEq/L (preop 134), potassium 4.5 mEq/L. Bun 12 mg/dl, creatinine 1.2 mg/dl. Serum osmolarity 286 mOsm/kg H_2O.

Question: What syndrome is this patient exhibiting?

Diagnosis: Transurethral prostatectomy (TURP) syndrome

Discussion: It is estimated that 2% of prostatic resections are complicated by TURP syndrome. TURP syndrome generally is believed to be the result of acute water intoxication leading to hypervolemia and dilutional hyponatremia. The symptom complex lacks a consistent presentation and varies in degree of seriousness from mildly symptomatic to death. The stereotypical presentation is that of nausea, confusion, bradycardia, and hypertension followed by hypotension. Profound hyponatremia consistently is found. The patient may complain of blurred vision or blindness. Respiratory distress or seizures may develop. In the most serious cases, coma or death may occur.

The pathophysiology of TURP syndrome is complex. Not all symptoms are easily explained. However, most researchers agree that the syndrome is the result of acute water intoxication and dilutional hyponatremia from absorption of irrigating fluid. Fluid is absorbed either through venous sinuses opened during the resection or via the periprostatic and retroperitoneal space if there is extravasation of fluid due to breach in the capsule. Initially, there is hypervolemia and hypertension leading to reflex bradycardia. Profound dilutional hyponatremia occurs, often with serum sodium less than 120 mEq/L, which implies absorption of 3–4 L of fluid. Hypertension then is followed by a "shock-like" leakage of water from plasma to the interstitium, resulting in hypotension and pulmonary edema.

The most common irrigating fluid used today is hypotonic 1.5% glycine (200 mmol/L) solution. Glycine solution is used because it is electrically inert and near isotonic with plasma, and allows clear visibility. Glycine is a nonessential amino acid that is metabolized by oxidative deamination to glyoxylic acid and ammonia. Hyperglycinemia and hyperammonemia have been implicated in causing many symptoms of the syndrome. Glycine may act as an inhibitory neurotransmitter at the retina to cause transient visual disturbances. Hyperammonemia is thought to cause many of the other CNS disturbances.

The symptoms of the dilutional hyponatremia are related to the speed of its development. Acute changes are thought to cause more profound symptoms and cerebral edema. The calculated osmolality—$2x$ (Na) + (glucose) + (urea)—often is lower than the measured osmolality (which is determined by freezing point depression), giving an osmolar gap greater than 10 mosm/kg. This osmolar gap indicates the presence of the solute glycine and its metabolites. It seems that the most serious cases are the result of a hyposmolar hyponatremia with a small osmolar gap.

Several risk factors for the development of TURP syndrome have been isolated. However, none seem to be of more importance than the experience of the surgeon and meticulous technique. Risk is thought to be increased in patients with a gland larger than 45 grams and/or resection time over 90 minutes. In addition, the height at which the irrigation fluid is hung (if greater than 60 centimeters) may lead to greater fluid absorption and thus greater risk. Some have argued that the use of a spinal anesthetic may increase risk of a more profound hypotension if TURP syndrome should occur. However, most anesthesiologists agree that a spinal allows close monitoring of the patient's mental status and, therefore, avoidance of severe TURP syndrome.

The treatment of TURP syndrome is somewhat controversial and lacks a clear consensus. However, most would agree that if the patient is mildly symptomatic and hemodynamically stable, monitoring and observation are sufficient until resolution of symptoms. If evidence of fluid overload exists (i.e., pulmonary edema), a loop diuretic may be appropriate. In the severely symptomatic patient who is comatose or having seizures, infusion of 200 cc of 3% hypertonic saline over 4 hours may be of clinical value. Some have argued, however, that hypertonic saline may exacerbate pre-existing pulmonary edema. The most feared complication of rapid correction of hyponatremia is the development of central pontine myelinolysis. Therefore, hypertonic saline infusion should be reserved for the severely symptomatic. Treatment should be aimed at raising serum sodium concentration at a rate of 1 mmol/hr until the patient becomes alert and symptom-free.

Prevention of TURP syndrome is aimed at limiting the amount of free water absorbed during the resection. Therefore, most urologists limit their resection time to less than 90 minutes and keep the irrigating fluid bag no higher than 60 centimeters. In addition, fluid absorption, serum sodium, and central venous pressure are monitored to avoid excess fluid absorption. Some institutions have employed tracer amounts of ethanol in the irrigating fluid which then can be detected in the expired breath to reflect the degree of dilutional hyponatremia.

In summary, TURP syndrome is a potentially deadly complication of excessive absorption of irrigating fluid. The syndrome can be avoided by awareness of the pathophysiology and vigilance in limiting irrigating fluid absorption.

In the present patient, TURP syndrome was suspected because of the change in mental status, change in hemodynamics, and evidence of fluid overload on exam (bibasilar crackles). The diagnosis was confirmed by the serum sodium of 120 mEq/L and the absence of other possible etiologies such as hypoxia, drug reaction, and hypoglycemia. The first priority was to secure the airway and stabilize the patient hemodynamically. The patient was conscious and stable, without seizures. He received Lasix 20 mg IV and was observed. The patient responded and diuresed nicely, with complete resolution of symptoms over the next 4 hours.

Clinical Pearls

1. It is estimated that 2% of prostatic resections are complicated by TURP syndrome.
2. TURP syndrome is the result of acute water intoxication and dilutional hyponatremia from absorption of irrigating fluid.
3. Glycine solution (1.5%) is a common irrigant because it is electrically inert and near isotonic, and allows for a clear visual field.
4. Glycine may directly inhibit the retina, causing visual disturbances.
5. A prostate gland larger than 45 grams or resection time greater than 90 minutes may increase the risk of TURP syndrome.

REFERENCES

1. Rao PN: Fluid absorption during urological endoscopy. Br J Urol 60:93–99, 1989.
2. Bernstein GT, Loughlin KR, Gittes RF: The physiologic basis of the TURP syndrome. J Surg Res 46:135–141, 1989.
3. Hahn RG: The transurethral resection syndrome. Acta Anaesthesiol Scand 35:557–567, 1991.
4. Jensen V: The TURP syndrome. Can J Anaesth 38:90–97, 1991.
5. Ayus JC, Arieff AL: Glycine-induced hypo-osmolar hyponatremia. Arch Intern Med 157:223–226, 1997.
6. Gravenstein D: Transurethral resection of the prostate (TURP) syndrome: A review of the pathophysiology and management. Anesth Analg 84:438–446, 1997.
7. Walsh P, Retik AB, Vaughan ED, Wein AJ (eds): Cambell's Urology, 7th ed. Philadelphia, W.B. Saunders and Company, 1998.

PATIENT 36

A 61-year-old man with a painless ulcer on the glans penis

A 61-year-old man presents with a chief complaint of a painless ulcer on the glans penis. He first noted the lesion 8 months ago, but recently it has grown significantly and has a whitish discharge. Otherwise he has no complaints and takes only a "pill for my blood pressure." The patient has had sexual contact only with his wife of 39 years.

Physical Examination: General: slightly obese, healthy-appearing. Temperature 37.6°; unremarkable vital signs. Chest and abdomen: normal. Genitalia: phimosis; 3-cm, shallow, erythematous ulceration on left, dorsal surface of glans; no urethral discharge; 1-cm, firm, nontender, and freely movable nodule in right groin. Rectal exam: normal.

Laboratory Findings: CBC, biochemistry profile: normal. Cultures of ulcer and urethra: negative.

Question: What is the most likely diagnosis?

Diagnosis: Carcinoma of the penis

Discussion: The differential diagnosis for a penile ulceration includes: (1) sexually transmitted diseases, such as syphilis, chancroid, or genital herpes; (2) trauma; (3) premalignant lesions, such as leukoplakia or balanitis; (4) carcinoma in situ, such as Bowen's disease or erythroplasia of Queyrat; and (5) invasive carcinoma, usually squamous cell, but basal cell and melanoma occur rarely.

Malignant lesions of the penis are uncommon, and they almost invariably are squamous cell carcinoma. Squamous cell lesions of the penis account for 0.4% of all cancers in the United States, with a stable incidence over the last 25 years. This malignancy is more common in other populations and is responsible for up to 15% of malignancies in some areas of India, Africa, and South America.

The etiology of penile squamous cell carcinoma is similar to lesions in other parts of the body—namely, chronic irritation. In particular, poor hygiene and smegma have been implicated in the process. Chronic inflammation secondary to debris trapped under the foreskin may be the mechanism of malignant degeneration. In support of this theory, neonatal circumcision virtually eliminates the disorder. Interestingly, adult circumcision does not provide the same immunity. In one study, 9% of patients with penis cancer had circumcision prior to developing carcinoma. Infection also has been invoked as a possible etiology. Human papilloma virus DNA has been isolated from half of studied populations with penile cancer, and has been shown to be associated with other neoplasms. Given these possible causative factors, it is not surprising that lack of circumcision, the presence of phimosis, advancing age, and concurrent venereal disease are all risk factors. The incidence increases with age, with the average age at presentation being 60 years old. However, there is a wide age range, and penile carcinomas have been documented as early as the second decade.

Characteristic morphologies include exophytic and ulcerative. The exophytic lesions tend to be better differentiated, while the ulcerative lesions are more common and have a worse prognosis. Ulceration, which occurs in 85% of cases, often is complicated by infection. Infection frequently is characterized by a discharge or reactive lymphadenopathy, which typically is what brings the patient to medical attention. It is important to note the high incidence of inflammatory lymphadenopathy: 60% of patients present with clinically positive (palpable) nodes, but only half of these have biopsy-proven nodal disease.

The heralding lesion is usually a small lump or ulcer, most often confined to the penis. In about 50% of patients, initial lesions are located on the glans. The prepuce is the next most common site. Lesions originating on the shaft account for the remainder. Sixty percent of lesions are less than 2 centimeters at presentation. The presence of phimosis may delay diagnosis until pain, bleeding, discharge, or obstruction evolve. Because of this variety in presentation, the importance of tissue biopsy cannot be understated. A high clinical index of suspicion is needed, and empiric therapy for a presumed infectious or dermatologic diagnosis should not delay biopsy.

Workup should include a careful history and physical examination, with attention to palpation of the groin for inguinal lymphadenopathy. Patients with ulceration complicated by infection or hemorrhage may have a leukocytosis or anemia. Along with biopsy, cultures and serologic tests can help to rule out other possible etiologies. Chest radiograph, bone scan, and computed tomography of the abdomen and pelvis are useful for metastatic evaluation in selected cases.

Buck's fascia is a potent barrier to invasion of the corpora and subsequent hematogenous dissemination. Only 2% of patients have initial hematogenous spread without prior nodal involvement. The lungs are the most likely site, but bone, liver, and brain also can be involved. The lymphatics are a much more common route of metastasis, primarily to the femoral and iliac nodes. There is a great deal of confluence in the lymphatic drainage of the penis, so bilateral and contralateral lymphadenopathy are common. Regional node disease frequently is the cause of death in penile cancer patients, either because of sepsis secondary to ulceration or hemorrhage secondary to erosion into the femoral vessels.

Prognosis correlates with presence of nodes, tumor stage, tumor location, vascular invasion, and loss of blood-group (ABO) antigens. Nodal status is by far the most important for predicting outcome and directing treatment. Several staging schemes exist, of which the most commonly used is the Jackson system. **Stage I** consists of primary tumors limited to the glans or prepuce, which carry an excellent prognosis. **Stage II** includes locally invasive disease involving the corpora cavernosa without nodal disease. Overall, stage I and II 5-year survival is 85%. **Stage III** includes clinically positive nodal involvement, and **stage IV** denotes spread beyond the penis to neighboring structures or distant metastasis. Five-year survival drops off to 50% with positive nodes, and is much lower for metastatic disease. Tumor grade also is an important predictor of metastasis, with nodal or distant spread in 15%

of patients with low-grade disease versus 40–80% with moderate or high-grade disease. The vast majority of the mortality associated with penile carcinoma occurs within 5 years of diagnosis.

Treatment strategies depend on the tissue diagnosis and extent of disease. A primary goal of therapy is to preserve the integrity and function of the organ, especially the ability to direct the urine stream. For reliable patients with in situ disease, topical bleomycin or fluorouracil and close followup is acceptable. Lesions solely involving the prepuce can be treated adequately with circumcision alone. Nd-YAG laser treatments also are used to treat local disease.

For invasive carcinoma, radiation therapy and surgical resection are the major options. Surgical resection—a partial or total penectomy—with adequate (2 centimeter) margins is the definitive therapy. Penectomy is associated with a 10% risk of local recurrence. Of these patients with negative nodes, 14% will become clinically positive, usually within 36 months. Lesions of the glans or prepuce treated with local resection have a 25% recurrence rate, and need especially careful followup.

Although penile cancer is primarily a surgical disease, radiotherapy can be useful for localized, low-grade lesions. Five-year survival in selected node-negative patients has been 70–80%. Radiation is attractive because it avoids mutilation of the penis, but it also carries a three-fold greater risk of local recurrence. In these patients, penectomy almost always is effective for salvage therapy. Salvage penectomy also can be necessary in up to 15% of irradiated patients because of side effects such as urethral stenosis or radiation necrosis. Finally, a post-treatment biopsy should be obtained to document tumor eradication.

For clinically evident nodal disease, an important first step is a 4- to 6-week course of broad-spectrum antibiotic therapy, because more than half of palpable lymphadenopathy is reactive or inflammatory. Patients with corporal, urethral, or vascular invasion or high-grade tumor are at risk for positive nodes and should have a prophylactic lymphadenectomy. All patients with persistently enlarged nodes also should have a lymph node dissection. The classic lymphadenectomy takes the lymphatic tissue from the sartorius laterally to the adductor longus medially and from 2 centimeters above the inguinal ligament to the apex of the femoral triangle inferiorly. Flap necrosis, debilitating edema, and wound infection are among significant morbidities that occur postoperatively in a small percentage of patients. Less extensive dissections have been proposed to further reduce this complication rate without sacrificing survival.

Effective therapies for systemic disease are still being developed. Currently, regimens of fluorouracil, cisplatinum, and bleomycin most commonly are used.

In the present patient, a biopsy of the glans lesion revealed squamous cell carcinoma. He was treated with a 2-week course of broad-spectrum antibiotics, and his lymphadenopathy resolved. He then underwent partial penectomy, with an uncomplicated hospital course. After his initial followup visits for wound care, the patient will be followed annually for recurrence surveillance.

Clinical Pearls

1. The diagnosis of carcinoma of the penis requires high clinical suspicion and tissue biopsy.

2. Squamous cell carcinoma is responsible for the overwhelming majority of penile tumors.

3. Penis cancer is primarily a disease of older, uncircumcised men.

4. Lymphadenopathy is common at presentation, but is benign in 50% of patients.

5. The definitive therapy is surgical resection.

6. Indications for lymphadenopathy include invasive or high-grade disease, as well as persistently palpable nodes after a curse of antibiotic therapy. Prophylactic lymphadenectomy in moderate-grade, localized disease remains controversial.

REFERENCES

1. Sufrin G, Huben R: Benign and malignant lesions of the penis. In Gillenwater JY, Grayhack JT, Howards SS, Duckett JW (eds): Adult and Pediatric Urology. St. Louis, Mosby, 1996, pp 1997–2042.
2. Adeyosu AB, Thornhill J, Corr J, et al: Prognostic factors in squamous cell carcinoma of the penis and implications for management. Br J Urol 80(6):937–939, 1997.
3. Pizzocaro G, Piva L, Bandieramonte G, Tana S: Up-to-date management of carcinoma of the penis. Eur Urol 32(1):5–15, 1997.

PATIENT 37

A 4-year-old girl with hydronephrosis

A 4-year-old girl presents with hydronephrosis. She has a history of recurrent febrile and afebrile urinary tract infections. The mother notes that a prenatal ultrasound revealed "a swollen kidney." The patient has no other significant past medical history and is not currently on any medications.

Physical Examination: Vital signs: normal. Abdomen: soft, nontender, nondistended, no palpable masses. Back: no palpable or visible sacral abnormalities. Genitalia: typical for 4-year-old female, no discharge. Rectum: normal.

Laboratory Findings: Urine dip stick: pH 6, leukocyte +2, blood +2, protein trace. Renal and bladder ultrasound: right-sided grade 2/4 hydronephrosis, area in upper pole consistent with scarring; normal echotexture on left, no evidence of hydronephrosis; distended, smooth-walled bladder, 180 cc capacity; ureters not visualized.

Question: What further imaging studies are indicated?

Diagnosis: Vesicoureteral reflux, right, grade 2

Discussion: Hydronephrosis is the most common congenital anomaly detected by prenatal ultrasound, and it represents 50% of all prenatally detected conditions. The majority of hydronephrosis detected in utero is physiologic and resolves by the end of pregnancy or within 1 year of age. The initial evaluation of a neonate with prenatally detected hydronephrosis should consist of an ultrasound within the first few days of life. Neonatal oliguria can mask significant pathology, and if an ultrasound performed within the first 48 hours of birth is negative, a repeat study is warranted at 4 weeks of age.

In order to standardize the grading system for hydronephrosis, the Society for Fetal Urology devised a 0–4 grading system. Based upon the long axis view of the kidney, this classification takes into account the degree to which the renal pelvis splits the central complex, the amount of calyceal dilatation, and the loss of parenchyma. In a 4-year-old girl, the differential diagnosis of hydronephrosis includes vesicoureteral reflux, ureteropelvic junction obstruction, ureterocele, duplication anomaly, megaureter, and ectopic ureter.

Voiding cystourethrography is warranted in all cases of hydronephrosis. Vesicoureteral reflux may coexist with a ureteropelvic or ureterovesical junction obstruction in 14% of patients. A **diuretic renogram** is warranted to assess function and drainage of a markedly hydronephrotic kidney. The renogram allows analysis of split differential renal function as well as evaluation of the washout curves. However, the lower glomerular filtration rate, poor concentrating ability, and variable response to furosemide in the newborn indicate the pitfalls of complete reliance on the diuretic renogram to diagnose obstruction in the newborn. The **intravenous pyelogram** is an excellent anatomic study with a functional component; however, gaseous distention of the bowel and poor concentrating ability of the kidney limit its usefulness in the newborn. The Whitaker antegrade pressure-flow perfusion study attempts to quantify obstruction in the dilated kidney. It is based on the premise that a high renal pelvic pressure, in relation to bladder pressure, documents an obstructive process. It records the response of the renal pelvis to distention, but this may not truly define obstruction in all cases. Moreover, the Whitaker study is invasive and requires anesthesia. Thus, it is no longer commonly employed.

The overwhelming majority of infants with prenatally detected hydronephrosis that is confirmed postnatally should be placed on prophylactic antibiotic pending a thorough evaluation. In the neonate, amoxicillin is an appropriate first-line prophylactic antibiotic. By 2 months of age, amoxicillin can be replaced with trimethoprim-sulfamethoxazole, which achieves excellent urinary concentration.

In the present patient, an ultrasound had not been performed within the first few days of life, though hydronephrosis had been detected prenatally. Current performance of voiding cystourethrography revealed a grade 2 vesicoureteral reflux. A diuretic renogram suggested a nonobstructing pattern. She was placed on prophylactic antibiotics and given a trial of observation with serial urine analyses.

Clinical Pearls

1. Hydronephrosis is the most common congenital anomaly detected by prenatal ultrasound.

2. The initial evaluation of a neonate with prenatally detected hydronephrosis should consist of an ultrasound within the first few days of life.

3. A voiding cystourethrogram is warranted in *all* cases of hydronephrosis.

4. Vesicoureteral reflux may coexist with a ureteropelvic or ureterovesical junction obstruction in 14% of patients.

REFERENCES
1. Conway JJ, Maizels M: The "well tempered" diuretic renogram: A standard method to evaluate the asymptomatic neonate with hydronephrosis or hydroureteronephrosis. J Nuc Med 33:2047–2051, 1992.
2. Blyth B, Snyder H, Duckett J: Antenatal diagnosis and subsequent management of hydronephrosis. J Urol 149:693–698, 1993.
3. Fernbach S, Maizels M, Conway J: Ultrasound grading of hydronephrosis: Introduction to the system used by the Society for Fetal Urology. Pediatr Radiol 23:478–479, 1993.

PATIENT 38

A newborn male with the urethral opening on the underside of his penis

A newborn male was born with a developmental anomaly affecting his urethral meatus. The mother (G3P3) had an uneventful prenatal course. There is no history of infertility, consanguinity, ingestion of medications during pregnancy, or family members with genital anomalies. There are two healthy male siblings. The baby voided through the penoscrotal meatus during examination.

Physical Examination: Vital signs: normal. General appearance: no dysmorphic features. Abdomen: soft, nontender, nondistended, no palpable masses. Genitalia: testicles bilaterally nonpalpable; urethral opening located at junction of penis and scrotum, severe chordee and dorsal hood; stretched penile length 3 centimeters; no hyperpigmentation of scrotum, urethral meatus in the upper midline. Back: no palpable sacral anomalies.

Laboratory Findings: CBC: normal. Electrolytes: normal. Buccal smear: equivocal. Karyotype: 46, XY.

Question: What diagnostic studies are indicated to confirm the diagnosis?

Diagnosis: Penoscrotal hypospadias with undescended testicles

Discussion: A newborn with hypospadias and cryptorchidism should be considered as having an intersex disorder until proved otherwise. Initial evaluation should begin with a thorough family history with regards to perinatal or neonatal deaths, consanguinity, and infertility. Maternal history—especially any drug or alcohol ingestion or hormone administration (progestational agents) during pregnancy—needs to be evaluated. Chromosomal analysis is accomplished by formal karyotyping in lieu of the buccal smear, which can be inaccurate. Biochemical evaluation is directed at ruling out congenital adrenal hyperplasia—specifically the salt-wasting variety, which may prove life-threatening. This is accomplished by measuring the plasma 17-hydroxyprogesterone level or via a 24-hour urine test for 17-ketosteroids and pregnanetriol.

The physical examination should begin with simple observation, looking for any dysmorphic features. The stretched penile length is measured along the dorsum of the phallus from the tip of the glans to the pubic ramus. The phallus is evaluated for the degree of chordee, location of the urethral meatus, and possibility of a urogenital sinus. The scrotum is assessed for the degree of fusion and the presence of testicles. A gonad palpated below the inguinal ligament is a testes until proven otherwise. Genital hyperpigmentation may be present, as with congenital adrenal hyperplasia.

Imaging studies include an ultrasound as well as a genitogram. Sonographic evaluation may be helpful in detecting a uterus or ovaries, and a genitogram delineates the internal anatomy and detects the presence of mullerian structures. The presence of testicles can be determined via laparoscopy or with a provocative human chorionic gonadotropin (HCG) stimulation test.

In the present patient, the chromosomal analysis revealed 46, XY. He is a normal male with undescended testicles bilaterally and penoscrotal hypospadias. The presence of testicular tissue was documented with a HCG test, and the 17-hydroxyprogesterone was normal. The penoscrotal hypospadias will be treated after 6 months of age and prior to the first birthday. Due to the severe amount of chordee, the child may require a staged repair, which may include a dermal graft to correct the chordee.

Clinical Pearls

1. A newborn with bilaterally undescended testicles or even unilateral undescended testicles with hypospadias should be considered an intersex patient until proved otherwise.
2. A gonad palpated below the inguinal ligament is a testicle until proved otherwise.
3. Formal karyotyping should be used to definitively determine chromosomal sex.
4. Serum 17-hydroxyprogesterone levels are analyzed or 24-hour urine 17-ketosteroids and pregnanetriol levels are used to evaluate the patient for congenital adrenal hyperplasia.
5. With bilaterally, nonpalpable testes, the presence of functioning testicular tissue must be verified.

REFERENCES
1. Rajfer J, Walsh PC: The incidence of intersexuality in patients with hypospadias and cryptorchidism. J Urol 116:769–770, 1976.
2. Donahue P, Powell D, Lee M: Clinical management of intersex abnormalities. Curr Probl Surg 28:513–579, 1991.

PATIENT 39

A 4-year-old boy with flank pain and hematuria

A 4-year-old boy presented with mild left flank pain and gross hematuria after falling off of a swing. There is no past medical or surgical history, although the parents state that he has complained of periodic, vague left abdominal pain.

Physical Examination: Vital signs: normal. Abdomen: soft, nondistended; mild tenderness and fullness in left upper quadrant. Testes: bilaterally descended, normal to palpation. Phallus: circumcised. Back: no palpable or visible sacral abnormalities.

Laboratory Findings: Urine culture: no growth. Urinalysis: specific gravity 1.020, pH 5, red blood cells 25–50, white blood cells 0–2. Radiograph of kidneys, ureter, and bladder: negative for calcifications, nonspecific bowel gas pattern. Renal and bladder ultrasound: grade 3 left hydronephrosis, grade 0 right hydronephrosis. Calculated bladder capacity: 200 cc. Post-void residual: 3 cc. Diuretic renogram: left differential renal function 33%, right 67%. Left T1/2 = 33 minutes, right T1/2 = 4 minutes. Voiding cystourethrogram: normal.

Question: What are the pitfalls of the tests screening for a ureteropelvic junction obstruction?

Diagnosis: Left ureteropelvic junction obstruction

Discussion: Impediment to the flow of urine from the renal pelvis into the ureter is referred to as a ureteropelvic junction obstruction (UPJO). It arises most commonly from an intrinsic lesion (e.g., narrowing, excess collagen deposition, ureteral valves, ureteral polyps) at the ureteropelvic junction. Other causes include extrinsic factors such as aberrant, crossing vessels or secondary obstruction from vesicoureteral reflux. A great deal of debate exists concerning what constitutes obstruction—even when diuretic renography is employed for clarification.

In the pre-ultrasound era, an abdominal mass, pain, sepsis, or urinary tract infections were among the common presenting signs and symptoms for a UPJO. However, maternal ultrasonography has resulted in the widespread diagnosis of asymptomatic, upper tract dilatation. It is now evident that all dilatation does not represent significant obstruction. Because of the morphologic appearance of a UPJO prenatally, the dilemma of when and if to intervene remains a point of controversy. Some investigators have shown that early intervention is effective in allowing the affected kidney to regain function. However, others have shown that little deterioration in renal function occurs in children with moderate obstruction who are followed conservatively. In the newborn who has a kidney with an apparent UPJO, an initial conservative, nonoperative approach with interval ultrasounds as well as renal scans appears to be a reasonable approach. Ultimately, the goal is to preserve renal function.

In the past, an intravenous pyelogram was the initial screening study. It provided an excellent anatomic picture of the ureteropelvic junction and what was considered an obstructive pattern. The intravenous pyelogram has been superseded by renal ultrasound and the diuretic renogram. The diuretic renogram attempts to objectify a subjective diagnosis. The degree of tracer uptake and the washout curves are intended to quantify function as well as obstruction. However, pitfalls including a lower glomerular filtration rate in the newborn, poor concentrating ability, and variable response to furosemide limit the usefulness of the study. The Whitaker antegrade pressure-flow perfusion study attempts to quantify obstruction in the dilated kidney. It is based on the premise that a high renal pelvic pressure, in relation to bladder pressure, documents an obstructive process. It records the response of the renal pelvis to distention, but this may not truly define obstruction in all cases. Also, this study is invasive and requires anesthesia.

There are a number of well described and time-honored repairs for UPJO, including approaches through the flank and the posterior lumbotomy. It is worthwhile for the surgeon to fully image the ureter prior to surgery in order to locate the level of the obstruction and exclude any concomitant ureteral pathology. A voiding cystourethrogram, to exclude coexisting vesicoureteral reflux, always is justified. The overwhelming majority of patients have a dilated, extrarenal pelvis that is amenable to the standard dismembered repair. This involves excision of the diseased segment and reanastomosis of the ureter to the renal pelvis. For a high insertion of a ureter with a small extrarenal component, a YV-plasty can be employed. A retroperitoneal drain is required in all cases.

As with many surgical techniques, anecdotal experiences weigh heavily on whether or not to stent. The choice of stents varies from the completely indwelling, internal catheter to the re-entry type catheter that acts as a nephroureteral stent and exits through the pelvis. A water-tight, spatulated, dependent repair is probably the single most important aspect in performing a pyeloplasty.

In the present patient, the clinical presentation along with grade 3 hydronephrosis and an obstructive pattern on renal scan strongly suggested a left ureteropelvic junction obstruction. Following a cystoscopy with retrograde pyelography, he underwent a stentless, dismembered pyeloplasty.

Clinical Pearls

1. An extrarenal pelvis must be distinguished from true pelvocalyceal dilatation.
2. A voiding cystourethrogram is warranted in all cases of UPJO to rule out coexisting reflux.
3. Neonatal pyeloplasty is not necessarily indicated when the affected kidney reveals good differential function.
4. There is no one ideal study to diagnose a UPJO.
5. A water-tight, spatulated, dependent repair is the single most important factor for a successful pyeloplasty.

REFERENCES

1. Homsy Y, Saad S, Laberge I, et al: Transitional hydronephrosis of the newborn and infant. J Urol 144:579–583, 1990.
2. Cartwright P, Duckett J, Keating M, et al: Managing apparent ureteropelvic junction obstruction in the newborn. J Urol 148:1224–1228, 1992.
3. Conway JJ, Maizels M: The "well tempered" diuretic renogram: A standard method to evaluate the asymptomatic neonate with hydronephrosis and hydroureteronephrosis. J Nuc Med 33:2047–2051, 1992.
4. Ducket JW: When to operate on neonatal hydronephrosis. Urology 42:617–619, 1993.
5. Macneily A, Maizels M, Kaplan W: Does early pyeloplasty really avert loss of renal function? A retrospective review. J Urol 150:769–773, 1993.

PATIENT 40

A 45-year-old woman with azotemia and bilateral flank masses

A 45-year-old woman with hypertension presents with the complaint of gradual onset of abdominal fullness and development of bilateral abdominal masses. The patient denies symptoms of flank pain, fever, gross hematuria, change in bowel habits, or other urinary symptoms. When asked about family history, she recalls her father dying of a myocardial infarction at age 60 after spending 3 years on dialysis. Her sister recently had surgery to clip a cerebral aneurysm. The patient denies any medication except for an antihypertensive.

Physical Examination: Afebrile, pulse 70, blood pressure 145/95. Chest: clear bilaterally. Cardiac: regular rate and rhythm, no murmurs. Back: no costovertebral tenderness. Abdomen: normoactive bowel sounds; nondistended; bilaterally palpable, nontender, irregular masses inferior to costal margins (right equals left); bladder nonpalpable. Genitalia: unremarkable.

Laboratory Findings: CBC normal. BUN 45 mg/dl, creatinine 3.2 mg/dl. Urinalysis: unremarkable, except for specific gravity of 1.0015. Renal ultrasound: markedly enlarged kidneys bilaterally; parenchyma largely replaced by numerous cysts of varying size; no obvious hydronephrosis (although difficult to assess given degree of cystic change); multiple small hepatic cysts incidentally noted.

Questions: What is the diagnosis? What are the unique management considerations in this urologic disorder?

Diagnosis: Autosomal dominant polycystic kidney disease (ADPKD)

Discussion: ADPKD is the most common cause of cystic changes within the kidney, and it is the etiology of end-stage renal disease in approximately 10% of dialysis patients. As the name implies, ADPKD is a genetic disorder that has been linked to mutations on both chromosomes 16 and 4. Autosomal dominant inheritance results in a 50% chance of affliction for children of an affected parent, but the disorder has variable penetrance and age of onset. Approximately 25% of patients with ADPKD have no family history and therefore either represent spontaneous mutations, or their affected parent failed to live long enough to manifest the disease.

Patients with ADPKD enjoy normal renal function and anatomy for the first 10 years of life. Moving into the second decade, however, the anatomic perturbations begin to develop despite virtually all patients remaining asymptomatic until about 30 years of age. Typically between the ages of 30–40, patients begin to experience symptoms of pain, hematuria, or urinary tract infection as the number and size of cysts progress. Most people maintain near normal renal function until the fifth decade, at which time both BUN and creatinine begin to rise. Even prior to development of renal insufficiency there is evidence of a defect in the kidney's ability to concentrate urine. The onset of renal insufficiency, as measured by elevated creatinine, represents a late manifestation of ADPKD. Renal deterioration is rapid, with roughly 50% of people suffering end-stage renal disease by the age of 60.

There are multiple anomalies associated with ADPKD, many of which are cystic in nature. **Hepatic cysts** are seen in approximately 50% of patients, and, although liver function is not impaired, the size of the cysts can be massive such that the patient may manifest symptoms solely from mass effect. Early satiety, nausea, and reflux are all common in patients with substantial hepatic involvement. In addition, the pancreas, ovaries, spleen, and subarachnoid space are subject to possible cystic change in ADPKD. Perhaps the most ominous associated anomalies are **intracranial aneurysms**. As many as 40% of patients may have asymptomatic intracranial lesions, and the average age at which these rupture in the ADPKD patient is much earlier than in the general population. There appears to be a subset of patients with ADPKD and aneurysms; therefore, it is recommended that ADPKD patients with a family history of known aneurysms or acute cerebrovascular accident should be screened, and those with identified lesions should undergo surgical treatment. Lastly, there also is a noted association with **cardiac valvular abnormalities** in ADPKD.

The parenchyma in kidneys affected by this disorder is replaced by hundreds of cysts ranging from millimeters to centimeters in diameter. These cysts are lined by cuboidal or columnar epithelium and can involve the nephron anywhere along its length. At their conception the cysts arise from the renal tubule, but as they increase in size their continuity with the tubule is lost, and they become isolated cystic structures.

Symptomatology in ADPKD is complex and often difficult to evaluate. Pain is the most common presenting symptom and usually precedes the development of a palpable renal unit. The character of pain is important in that a dull sensation is caused by the mass effect of the enlarged kidneys, possibly stretching the renal capsule or placing pressure on nearby organs. Acute pain usually signifies cyst rupture, infection, hemorrhage, colic secondary to clots or stones, or obstruction from cyst compression. Hematuria also is common and can signify cyst rupture as well as the more traditional causes, such as stones, infections, and neoplasms.

Evaluation of symptoms in ADPKD requires special consideration because imaging studies often fail to accurately diagnose, largely due to the massive distortion of the renal anatomy. CT with enhancement is the most useful imaging technique, as it allows for evaluation of possible infection, hemorrhage, and calculus disease. Ultrasound also is valuable; however, cyst calcification and massive cystic change make this tool less effective for evaluation of nephrolithiasis and hydronephrosis. Use of intravenous pyelography is limited as many of these patients have renal insufficiency, but it may help to localize the level of ureteral obstruction. CT, however, remains the most useful modality because it can best differentiate cysts from dilated calyces and can localize infection with better accuracy than alternative imaging techniques.

Infection requires additional discussion with regard to ADPKD. More than half of the patients with this disease suffer from urinary tract infections, and the vast majority of these infections occur in females. In fact, urine cultures may be sterile, depending on the location of the infection. Neither an infected cyst (pyocyst) nor an infected obstructed calyx communicates with the urinary tract, and a clean midstream urine culture can be obtained. Therefore, additional evaluation with CT is necessary to rule out infection in the setting of a negative urine culture. Moreover, treatment of infection in the setting of ADPKD is associated with considerable morbidity and mortality, and it requires the use of a lipophilic antimicrobial and/or formal drainage. Instrumentation of the urinary tract in these patients should not be routine, because of the inherent risk of infection.

In the present patient, manifestations of the disease are typical. Management is limited to treatment of associated urologic diseases such as infection, stones, neoplasms, and hemorrhage. Progression to end-stage renal disease is likely and, as there is no treatment available to postpone this inevitability (except for a possible therapeutic effect of aggressive treatment for concomitant hypertension), dialysis and transplantation remain the endpoint for unfortunate patients with this genetic disorder.

Clinical Pearls

1. ADPKD, the most common cause of cystic renal disease, results from a single genetic defect on either chromosome 4 or 16. The defect is inherited in an autosomal dominant manner and is the third most common cause of end-stage renal disease.

2. Cystic change also is seen in the liver, pancreas, spleen, thyroid, ovaries, testes, pineal gland, and subarachnoid space.

3. Intracranial aneurysms are seen in up to 40% of patients with ADPKD, and they are susceptible to rupture at a much earlier age than those found in the general population.

4. Instrumentation of the urologic tract should be avoided, if possible, because of the risk of introducing infection.

5. The risk of renal cell carcinoma in patients with ADPKD is the same as that in the general population; however, those patients that go on to require dialysis have an increased risk of renal cell carcinoma due to the development of acquired renal cystic disease associated with dialysis.

REFERENCE
Lippert MC: Renal cystic disease. In Gillenwater JY, Grayhack JT, Howards SS, Duckett JW (eds): Adult and Pediatric Urology, 3rd ed. St. Louis, Mosby, 1996, pp 931–940.

PATIENT 41

A 35-year-old man with extreme abdominal pain

A 35-year-old man presents to the emergency department writhing in pain. He awoke 1 hour ago with excruciating right lower quadrant pain radiating to his testicle. He cannot find comfort in any position. He is otherwise healthy, with a history of mild asthma and seasonal rhinitis. He takes only albuterol and claritin, as needed.

Physical Examination: Temperature 37.3°; pulse 108; respirations 24; blood pressure 139/82. General: mildly obese; obvious distress. Abdomen: soft; normal bowel sounds; very mild right-sided tenderness, greater in upper than in lower quadrant. Genitalia: circumcised phallus; nonbloody meatus; nontender descended testes. Rectal: heme negative; small, firm prostate.

Laboratory Findings: WBC 10,600/μl, BUN 10 mg/dl, creatinine 1 mg/dl. Urinalysis: specific gravity 1.040, pH 5, RBC 50–100/hpf, no bacteria. CT scan of abdomen/pelvis without contrast: see figures.

Question: What is the proper diagnosis and management of this patient?

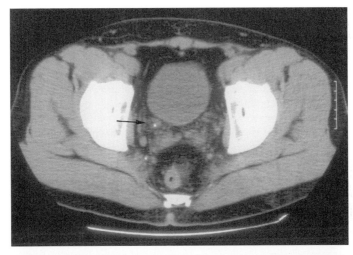

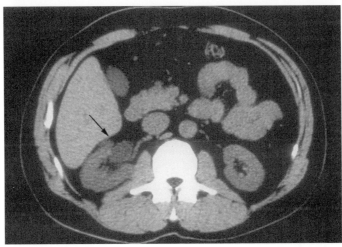

Diagnosis: Acute renal colic

Discussion: Renal colic is a commonly encountered diagnosis in the emergency department. Although often a classic presentation, it frequently is enigmatic and may be worked up as a surgical abdomen. The pain of colic is impressive. It is caused by the swelling of the renal capsule as well as calyceal and ureteral peristalsis against an obstructed urinary tract. This obstruction is caused almost invariably by stone; however, papillary necrosis (seen with diabetes, sickle cell, or phenacetin abuse), blood clots, congenital obstruction of the ureteropelvic junction, extrinsic compression, and aggregation of certain drugs can obstruct the ureter, as well.

The differential diagnosis can be vast, and which side the stone presents on can be critical. Acute appendicitis is the most frequent mimic in young patients. Bowel obstruction, pancreatitis, cholycystitis, gastroenteritis, diverticulitis, abdominal aortic aneurysm, and musculoskeletal etiologies should be ruled out. Testicular and ovarian pathologies also can present in a similar fashion.

Renal colic classically presents as sudden-onset, intense pain in the flank, groin, or testicle/labia, depending upon the level of the obstruction. The pain typically radiates down the ipsilateral side with intermittent waves. The patient usually is restless and unable to find a comfortable position. About 30% of patients present with gross hematuria. Because the kidney shares autonomic innervation with the gastrointestinal tract, nausea and vomiting almost always are present. Dehydration, often an inciting factor of renal colic, may be exacerbated by the vomiting. Nephrolithiasis is seen more commonly in the southwest and southeast United States, peaking in incidence during the summer months when dehydration is especially likely. Finally, any history of kidney stones is a strong predictor, as two thirds of patients will have recurrent stone formation.

Physical examination results are highly variable: low-grade fever, tachycardia, tachypnea, and elevated blood pressure are common. The abdomen is soft with mild tenderness on the affected side; however, the ileus becomes more prominent in protracted cases. Signs of frank peritonitis are rare, even when urine is extravasating from the collecting system. Patients often exhibit some degree of tenderness at the costovertebral angle.

Laboratory examination is very helpful. Gross or microhematuria is present in over 75% of patients. White cells also are seen, but generally not more than 10 per high-powered field. Urine pH may be helpful in determining the type of stone: acid pH suggests a uric acid stone, while alkaline pH suggests an infective or struvite stone. Other laboratory tests are less helpful, but a creatinine often is done to allow for the injection of IV contrast. Elevation may be a sign of underlying renal impairment and, thus, an indication for admission. It should be noted that the leukocyte count may be mildly elevated as a product of margination with an acute stressor; however, large elevations or a left shift are more indicative of possible active urinary tract infection. The latter is a strong indication for admission and/or intervention.

Oftentimes, the final diagnosis is not confirmed until a radiographic study is performed. Emergency departments today can easily obtain CT scans in an expeditious matter. However, a plain film of the kidneys, ureters, and bladder (KUB) will demonstrate 90–95% of all stones. Intravenous pyelography (IVP) is considered the gold standard, as it demonstrates the stone as well as the level and degree of obstruction, and can be used as a road map in the operating room. Unfortunately, IVP is falling out of favor because it tends to be a time-consuming and labor-intensive test, and it gives very little nonurologic information. Noncontrast CT has become the test of choice for many emergency department physicians. It is quick and highly sensitive for the detection of renal or ureteral calculi. In addition, it may identify other intra-abdominal pathology. Contrast can be added to the study to obtain functional information. If a delayed KUB is done after the infusion, a film similar to an IVP that demonstrates the level and degree of obstruction is obtained.

Once the diagnosis of stone is made, treatment can be initiated. The mainstays of treatment are vigorous hydration, adequate pain control, and urine straining. Admission is indicated only when several strict criteria are met: an inability to tolerate oral hydration, poor oral pain control, evidence of infection, solidary kidney, or significant renal impairment. Notably, not mentioned are: extravasation of urine, large stones, complete obstruction, or gross hematuria. An infected, obstructed urinary system is equivalent to an abscess, which requires urgent draining, either by percutaneous or endoscopic means.

Patients can be instructed to return in several days if their stone has not passed. The probability of passage is greatly dependent on size and location. Stones smaller than 5 millimeters pass in about 75% of cases, while stones greater than 8 millimeters pass less than 10% of the time. The stone obstructs at the three narrowest points: the ureteropelvic junction, the pelvic brim (where the iliac vessels cross the ureter), and the ureterovesicular junction (the narrowest). Once the stone has traversed these obstacles, passage should be imminent. It should be stressed to all patients that retrieval of the stone or stone fragments is imperative for analysis. Once the stone is characterized, significant steps can be taken to prevent recurrence. As a final note, patients may be assured that stones that do not pass almost always are amenable to a noninvasive approach, either extracorporeal shock-wave lithotripsy or endoscopic retrieval/manipulation.

In the present patient, renal colic presented classically: sudden-onset pain awoke him, radiated to his groin, and caused him to be uncomfortable in any position. The hematuria and the suggestive CT scan, which revealed a small ureteral calcification and right hydronephrosis, completed the diagnosis. The patient was treated expectantly with fluids and pain control measures. Unfortunately, he could not pass his stone, and it was retrieved endoscopically as an outpatient.

Clinical Pearls

1. Renal colic is characterized by sudden onset of intense pain in the flank, which often radiates to the groin or testicle.

2. Gross or microscopic hematuria is present in over 75% of patients.

3. KUB identifies 90% of stones, but a CT scan or IVP is needed to confirm the diagnosis.

4. Acute management consists of outpatient hydration and pain control. Admission is indicated in patients with compromised renal function, evidence of infection, or inability to tolerate outpatient management.

5. Obstructing stones in the face of infected urine is an emergency, requiring immediate drainage.

6. Urinary extravasation is inconsequential, not an operative indication.

REFERENCES
1. Abber JC, McAnnich JW: Renal colic: Emergency evaluation and management. Am J Emer Med 3:56–63, 1985.
2. Stewart C: Nephrolithiasis. Emer Med Clin N Am 6:617–630, 1988.
3. Platt JF: Urinary obstruction. Radiol Clin N Am 34:1113–1129, 1996.
4. Trivedi BK: Nephrolithiasis. PostGrad Med 100:63–78, 1996.
5. Begun FP, Foley WD: Patient evaluation laboratory and imaging studies. Urol Clin N Am 24:97–116, 1997.

PATIENT 42

A 30-year-old man with acute scrotal pain

A 30-year-old man presents to the emergency department with acute onset of pain in his left testicle about 5 hours ago. He is otherwise healthy, with no past medical history. He takes only aspirin for occasional headaches.

Physical Examination: Temperature 37.9°; pulse 99; respirations 22; blood pressure 139/82. General: obvious distress; patient lying on his right side. Abdomen: soft, nontender. Genitalia: circumcised phallus; markedly tender right testis; right epididymis.

Laboratory Findings: WBC 11,200/μl. BUN, creatinine: normal. Urinalysis: specific gravity 1.015, pH 5, WBC 5–8/hpf, RBC 3–5/hpf, 1+ bacteria. Duplex ultrasound: see figures.

Question: What is your next course of action?

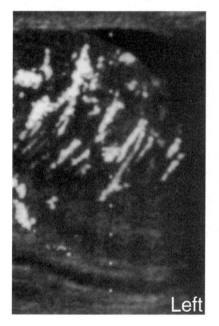 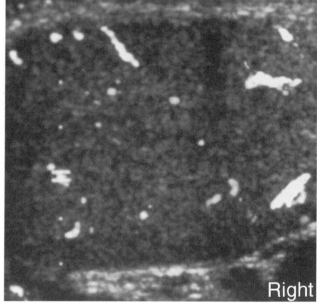

Diagnosis: Epididymitis

Discussion: The acute scrotum represents one of the few truly emergent urologic consultations. Indecisive action may result in the loss of a testicle and, frequently, litigation. Although this problem almost never is life-threatening, it is the source of high anxiety. The primary distinction that needs to be made in any case of acute scrotal pain is: **torsion versus nontorsion**. Age is a strong predictor of torsion; however, torsion always should be ruled out regardless of the patient's age.

The differential diagnosis for acute scrotal pain includes: torsion (torsion of the spermatic cord), epididymitis and/or orchitis, and torsion of the appendix testis. Also included, but less frequently, are: testicular tumor, hernia, varicocele with or without thrombus, Henoch-Schönlein purpura, Fourniers gangrene, idiopathic scrotal edema, and trauma. The first three entities account for well over 90% of cases. Furthermore, epididymitis is 10 times more common than torsion in the age group in question.

Torsion, more properly termed **torsion of the spermatic cord**, demands prompt attention. Certain details in the history, such as adolescent age, acute onset, nausea, vomiting, and a history of prior episodes, are particularly indicative of torsion. The left testicle is involved more frequently than the right, and the episode typically is preceded by a history of trauma, exercise, or sexual activity. Again, although 65% of cases occur between the ages of 12–18, this fact should never preclude the diagnosis. On physical exam the testis is very tender and may have an abnormally high, horizontal lie. In the past, Prehn's sign (temporary relief of pain by elevation of the scrotum) implied epididymitis. This sign now is largely discredited. However, if the physician can elicit the absence of the cremasteric reflex on the affected side, torsion is strongly suggested.

The definitive diagnosis of torsion frequently is made at the time of surgery. If a high clinical suspicion exists, there should be no hesitation to operate without further imaging. Much like appendicitis, a certain number of false positives are accepted to ensure the optimal rate of salvage. The rate of salvage approaches 97% if under 6 hours, 55–85% at 6–12 hours, 20–80% at 12–24 hours, and < 10% at more than 24 hours. Thus, it cannot be stressed enough that *time is of the essence*; with each passing hour, long-term results are dramatically affected. The treatment begins with manual detorsion, followed by immediate surgical exploration. The testis is examined carefully and removed if it is thought to be nonviable. If it is viable, an orchiopexy is performed bilaterally.

Oftentimes the **bell clapper deformity**—a congenital narrowing of the testicular attachment, predisposing to torsion—is seen, and the contralateral testicle is at high risk if not pexed.

If the diagnosis is too uncertain to proceed directly to surgery, further imaging should be obtained. The nuclear testicular scan, with an 88% or greater sensitivity, is thought to be the gold standard by many. However, it frequently is unavailable, especially after working hours. The Duplex ultrasound is more commonly used. This exam is highly operator-dependent. Some operators quote sensitivities of 82–100%. The hallmark is a heterogeneous testicle with absence of flow on Doppler interrogation.

Epididymitis is the most frequent cause of acute scrotal pain in post-adolescents. Pyuria (50%), fever (30%), and irritative voiding symptoms are strongly suggestive of the diagnosis. The presentation often is more chronic than acute, developing over the course of days. On physical exam, a tender, indurated epididymis often can be felt early in the course. Later, orchitis may make the testicle more tender, frequently with a reactive hydrocele. Epididymitis typically is caused by an infectious etiology. History is important in identification of causative agents, with heterosexual men presenting with chlamydia or gonorrhea. Homosexual men tend to be infected by coliforms and pseudomonas. The proper treatment involves prompt coverage for gonorrhea and chlamydia (e.g., intramuscular ceftriaxone and oral azithromycin) followed by a 10- to 14-day course of gram-negative coverage (e.g., quinolone). Of course, urine culture should be sent, and antibiotics tailored as indicated. Patients often find nonsteroidal anti-inflammatory drugs, bed rest, and scrotal support somewhat helpful.

Another common cause of acute scrotum is **torsion of testicular appendages**. Unlike testicular torsion, these are not treated with emergent detorsion. Torsion of the appendix testis or appendix epididymis is treated conservatively. These entities are classically seen in adolescents, but can appear at any age. They present with sudden pain that usually is milder than pain due to testicular torsion. Patients often can localize the pain to a specific point in the upper pole of their testis. The pathognomonic sign of appendicular torsion is the **blue dot sign**—a classically necrotic/cyanotic appendix testis seen on the upper pole of the otherwise normal testis.

Other, less frequently seen entities include: Fourniers gangrene (an aggressive, perineal, necrotizing fasciitis), testicular tumors (usually only seen acutely if there has been hemorrhage into the tumor), incarcerated hernia (a scrotal mass which frequently is accompanied by symptoms of intestinal obstruction), trauma (almost always obvious by history and the presence of ecchymoses), Henoch-Schönlein purpura (a systemic vasculitis seen in young children), varicocele (infrequently presents with acute pain unless there is acute thrombus), as well as a litany of other rare causes (e.g., Familial Mediterranean fever, venomous bites, cysticercosis). Almost all of these entities can be differentiated from the most common causes by a good history-taking and a thorough physical exam. The Doppler ultrasound should differentiate the more ambiguous cases.

In the present patient, a toxic appearance was absent. Additionally, he had pyuria and a markedly tender epididymis. Statistically, because of his age, epididymitis was likely. The ultrasound showed greatly increased blood flow to the affected side (*left figure*), consistent with epididymal orchitis. A short course of a fluoroquinolone and scrotal elevation cured this patient.

Clinical Pearls

1. Torsion is seen mostly in adolescents. It is acute in onset, and patients appear toxic and have a history of similar episodes.

2. The definitive diagnosis of torsion is made in the operating room. Time is of the essence.

3. Ultrasound and other imaging modalities are reserved for uncertain cases when timing is not as crucial.

4. Epididymitis is common in patients over 20 years old. It is marked by point tenderness, pyuria, fever, and irritative voiding symptoms. Gonorrhea, chlamydia, and gram-negative coliforms are the most common agents.

5. Torsion of the appendix testis is another common cause of acute scrotum. These patients appear much less toxic and may have the classic blue dot sign.

REFERENCES

1. Edelsberg JS, Surh YS: The acute scrotum. Emer Med Clin North Am 6:521–545, 1988.
2. Smith-Harrison LI, Koontz WW: Torsion of the testes: Changing concepts. AUA Update Series, Lesson 32, Vol IX:250–255, 1990.
3. Barloon TJ, Weissman AM, Kahn D: Diagnostic imaging of patients with acute scrotal pain. Am Fam Physician 53:1734–1750, 1996.
4. Siegel MJ: The acute scrotum. Radiol Clin North Am 35:959–976, 1997.

PATIENT 43

A 52-year-old woman with an incidentally discovered adrenal mass

A 52-year-old woman presents to the emergency department with the acute onset of right flank pain. The patient states that she has never had pain like this before. The pain radiates to the groin. She denies fever, chills, hematuria, and dysuria.

Physical Examination: General: writhing in pain. Pulse 96; blood pressure 160/100; respirations 18. Cardiac: regular rhythm and rate. Chest: clear to auscultation bilaterally. Abdomen: soft, nontender. Back: tenderness at right costovertebral angle. Pelvis: unremarkable.

Laboratory Findings: WBC 9600/μl, serum creatinine 1.2 mg/dl. Urinalysis: pH 7.0, RBC 11–50/hpf, WBC 0/hpf, no leukocyte esterase or nitrites. Noncontrast CT scan of abdomen and pelvis: 2 × 3 mm distal ureteral stone; 2 × 3 cm solid right adrenal mass.

Question: What workup, if any, should be performed for this incidentally discovered mass?

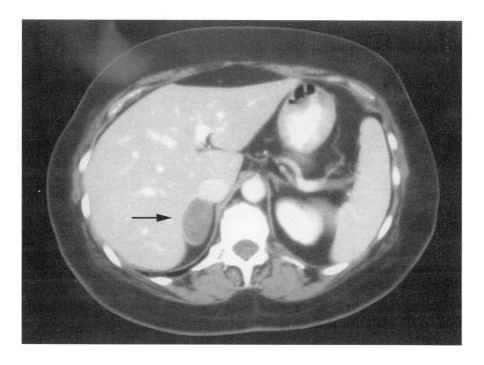

Diagnosis: Pheochromocytoma

Discussion: More prevalent use of abdominal CT, MRI, and ultrasound for various clinical problems has led to an increase in the diagnosis of "incidental" adrenal masses. The prevalence of these masses ranges from 0.6–1.3%.

The optimal evaluation of these patients remains controversial. Any evaluation must be selective and cost effective without sacrificing sensitivity and specificity. The workup of an incidental adrenal mass must determine whether it is benign or malignant and hormonally active or inactive. Therapeutic decisions regarding malignant lesions depend on whether the lesion is primary or metastatic. All tumors that demonstrate hormonal activity should be removed—regardless of histological findings.

There are several important considerations in the evaluation of the incidental adrenal mass, and these are not controversial. First, all patients with solid adrenal masses should undergo **endocrinologic evaluation**. If a biochemical perturbation is identified, it should be treated in the appropriate fashion. The actual algorithm for diagnosis of a hormonally active tumor varies from institution to institution.

The hormonal analysis should be tailored to the particular clinical features that exist in the involved patient. History and physical examination coupled with a minimal laboratory evaluation often can lead to a specific pathological diagnosis. Generally, the only automatic screen necessary is for pheochromocytoma, because of the great potential for morbidity related to this condition. Selectively screen for hyperaldosteronism in the hypertensive patient and for hypercortisolism in the patient who manifests the stigmata of Cushing's syndrome.

Pheochromocytoma, though rare, has particularly devastating consequences if not diagnosed. Therefore, *all patients with a solid adrenal mass should be evaluated for pheochromocytoma.* Clinical suspicion should be heightened in the patient who presents with hypertension, headache, and diaphoresis. All of these clinical findings are due to the physiological property of these tumors whereby they secrete catecholamines—dopamine, epinephrine, and norepinephrine. One review asserts that 93.8% of patients with pheochromocytoma have these symptoms. However, many other series show pheochromocytoma often are occult.

Generally, the hypertension is manifested as sustained baseline hypertension with additional paroxysms. Again, all patients with an incidental adrenal mass should be screened for pheochromocytoma—whether or not they are hypertensive. Pheochromocytoma have been known to cause cardiac dysrhythmias. Moreover, a number of these tumors can be found in association with hereditary disorders such as von Hippel-Lindau disease, MEN II A, and Sturge-Weber disease, as well as neurofibromatosis.

A reasonable screening regimen includes the determination of 24-hour urinary excretion of vanillylmandelic acid, metanephrines, and catecholamines. Tumors that secrete unmetabolized catecholamines are diagnosed with 24-hour urinary catecholamines. Those that excrete metabolized catecholamines are diagnosed with 24-hour urinary metanephrines. Approximately 95% of patients with pheochromocytoma have elevated levels of these markers.

Aldosterone-secreting adenoma accounts for 1% of hypertensive patients in the U.S., or 350,000 people. The hallmark of this entity is hypertension in the presence of hypokalemia. Aldosterone-secreting adenoma is infrequent in the normotensive population. Therefore, serum potassium levels as a screening tool should be used only in hypertensive patients with a mass. In hypertensive patients with spontaneous hypokalemia, specific hormonal testing should be undertaken to rule out an aldosterone-secreting adenoma. If the patient is normokalemic, the likelihood that an aldosterone-secreting tumor is present is rather small and does not warrant further screening.

Glucocorticoid-producing adenoma is extremely rare, particularly in the absence of clinical findings. If either hypertension or obesity is absent, the probability of finding a hormonally active mass is approximately 0.01%. Other clinical manifestations of excessive corticosteroids, such as easy bruisability, abdominal striae, moon facies, buffalo jump, or myopathy, increase the chance of the screening process yielding a positive result. Two or three 24-hour urine collections are recommended to look for elevated cortisol as a screening test for Cushing's syndrome.

Second, **surgical removal** should be performed on all nonfunctioning, solid lesions greater than 5 centimeters in size. This statement is based on the fact that most adrenal malignancies are greater than 6 centimeters, and the risk of malignancy increases with increasing size. Because of the potential for imaging to underestimate size of lesions, 5 centimeters has been considered in most circles to provide an excellent margin of safety. Those lesions that are smaller than 5 centimeters present a diagnostic dilemma. Most current recommendations center on obtaining an MRI to solve this problem. Adrenal carcinomas tend to be hypointense to the liver and spleen on T1-weighted images, and hyperintense to the liver and spleen on T2-weighted images. This is unlike adenomas, which appear hypointense on T1- and T2-weighted images. Those lesions that suggest carcinoma should be removed. Those suggestive of adenoma should be followed, with repeat imaging every 6 months. Any evidence of growth warrants repetition of screening tests to examine endocrine function and evaluate the necessity of lesion removal.

Cystic adrenal masses can be aspirated. Aspiration cytology should be analyzed by an experienced cytopathologist to evaluate for primary malignancy versus adenoma versus metastatic disease.

Treatment options for functional adrenal tumors generally involve surgical removal. Both open surgical and laparoscopic adrenalectomy can be used to remove these tumors. The choice of the approach depends on the size of the lesion (larger lesions are more amenable to open extirpation) and the preference of the surgeon. Adrenocortical carcinoma is treated with surgery. Even in the best circumstances, the prognosis for adrenal carcinoma is bleak. An adrenal mass that represents a metastatic lesion is best treated based on the current therapy for the primary lesion.

In the present patient, the stone ultimately passed spontaneously. Endocrinologic screening was performed for pheochromocytoma, and she had elevated 24-hour urinary catecholamines, consistent with this disorder. The urologist responsible for this patient consulted with an anesthesiologist familiar with the anesthetic management of this entity. The patient was admitted the evening before surgery and hydrated. Alpha adrenergic blockade was achieved prior to surgery. The patient underwent adrenalectomy, with extreme care taken to minimize manipulation of the affected adrenal gland. She tolerated the procedure well and is stable postoperatively.

Clinical Pearls

1. The endocrinologic evaluation of the incidentally discovered adrenal mass can be done selectively. All patients with an incidentally discovered adrenal mass should be screened for pheochromocytoma. Only hypertensive patients should be screened for hyperaldosteronism. Only those patients with the stigmata of Cushing's syndrome should be screened for hypercortisolism.

2. All solid tumors greater than 5 centimeters in size need to be resected, secondary to the risk of malignancy.

3. All metabolically active tumors should be resected.

4. All other adrenal tumors should be followed radiographically and, if interval growth is detected, re-evaluated metabolically and ultimately resected.

REFERENCES
1. Ross NS, Aron DC: Hormonal evaluation of the patient with an incidentally discovered adrenal mass. New Engl J Med 323:1401–1405, 1990.
2. Cook DM: Adrenal mass. Endocrinol Metab Clin North Am 26(4):829–852, 1997.
3. Vaughn ED Jr: Diagnosis of surgical adrenal disorders. AUA Update Series, Lesson 39, Vol XVI:306–311, 1997.

PATIENT 44

A 42-year-old woman with hypertension and an adrenal mass

A 42-year-old woman with no previous medical history presents to her internist with chief complaints of generalized muscle weakness, polyuria, and headache. She denies fever, chills, weight loss, night sweats, flushing, dysuria, and hematuria. She has no previous surgical history. She gave birth to two children over 10 years ago via normal, spontaneous, vaginal delivery; the pregnancies were full term and without complications. She reports a normal menstrual cycle. She takes no medications and denies tobacco, alcohol, and illicit drug use.

Physical Examination: Temperature 36.6°; pulse 72; respirations 12; blood pressure 170/100 without orthostatic changes. General: thin, no apparent distress. HEENT: mild retinopathy. Cardiac: regular rate and rhythm; no murmurs, gallops, or rubs. Abdomen: soft, without masses. Extremities: no cyanosis, clubbing, or edema.

Laboratory Findings: CBC normal. Sodium 147 mEq/L, potassium 3.2 mEq/L, bicarbonate 30 mEq/L. Thyroid function tests: normal. Urinalysis: pH 7.0, specific gravity 1.010, dipstick positive for mild protein, no RBC or WBC. ECG: normal sinus rhythm without T or Q wave abnormalities.

Question: What is the most likely diagnosis?

Diagnosis: Conn's syndrome

Discussion: Conn's syndrome is defined as adrenal hypersecretion of aldosterone in the hypertensive, nonedematous patient. It accounts for approximately 1% of the hypertensive patients in the United States (a remarkable 350,000 people!). Women with this diagnosis outnumber men by 2:1. The typical patient is 30–50 years old.

A clinical suspicion of primary hyperaldosteronism should be entertained in any hypertensive patient with spontaneous hypokalemia (serum potassium less than 3.5 mEq/L). The typical patient has muscle weakness (periodic paralysis at the extreme), polyuria, and headache. Headaches are due to hypertension. Muscle weakness, polyuria, and paresthesias relate to the effect of hypokalemia on skeletal muscle, the renal concentrating mechanism, and peripheral nerves, respectively. The major physical finding is hypertension without any evidence of peripheral edema. Funduscopic exam may show mild retinopathy. Lab analysis shows hypokalemia, dilute urine with pH greater than 6.5, elevated serum bicarbonate, and mild metabolic alkalosis. ECG often shows premature ventricular contractions, elevation of ST segments, and the presence of T and U waves.

A working knowledge of the renin-angiotensin-aldosterone axis is important to understand the metabolic abnormalities in Conn's syndrome. The critical sensor in this axis resides in the juxtaglomerular complex in the kidney. In response to a variety of stimuli, most commonly a fall in renal perfusion or decreased sodium intake, the plasma level of renin rises. This rise causes an increase in angiotensin I, angiotensin II, and, ultimately aldosterone. Aldosterone seeks to restore circulating blood volume. To achieve this end, aldosterone acts on the distal tubule and collecting ducts to cause the secretion of K^+ and, to a lesser extent, H^+ in exchange for Na. The retained sodium osmotically causes water to be reabsorbed into the body. This is the cause of the hypokalemic, hypernatremic, metabolic alkalosis seen in this entity.

A reasonable approach to the diagnosis of primary hyperaldosteronism is as follows. First, the patient must have hypertension and hypokalemia without any diuretic usage. Diuretic usage is the most common cause of hypokalemia in hypertensive patients. Additionally, other causes of hypertension, such as renal artery stenosis, can cause secondary hyperaldosteronism. This diagnosis is entertained in the patient with hypokalemia and hypertension in the setting of increased renin secretion, formation of angiotensin II, and subsequent aldosterone secretion. Additionally, anything that causes a compromise of renal blood flow and

activates the renin-angiotensin-aldosterone axis causes secondary hyperaldosteronism. Among these diagnoses are shock, pregnancy, and cirrhosis. Secondary hyperaldosteronism should be considered depending on the clinical circumstances.

If the above factors are absent, but hypertension and hypokalemia are present, the patient should be screened for primary hyperaldosteronism. However, some patients unconsciously realize that their weakness occurs with increased sodium intake. They restrict their sodium intake and by the renin-angiotensin-aldosterone axis they have normal potassium levels when observed. This entity should not be ruled out until the patient has adhered to a sodium-loading diet with 10 grams daily for several weeks and repeat potassium levels have been obtained. A few patients have normokalemic hyperaldosteronism, and they should be investigated further if the clinical suspicion is high.

Once the decision has been made to screen a particular patient, the test of choice is a paired random plasma aldosterone concentration (PAC)-to-plasma renin activity (PRA) ratio. A high ratio (greater than 20) indicates a positive screening test. These patients should be evaluated further for primary hyperaldosteronism. A high-sodium diet should be consumed for 3 days to help to suppress aldosterone secretion in those patients without primary hyperaldosteronism. Because the high-sodium diet can dramatically increase the excretion of potassium, potassium chloride supplementation is provided. After 3 days, a 24-hour urinary specimen for sodium and aldosterone should be obtained. If the sodium level exceeds 200 mEq/L, adequate sodium repletion is documented, and any aldosterone level obtained is a true value. If the aldosterone level exceeds 12 µg within 24 hours, a diagnosis of primary hyperaldosteronism is made.

At this point a CT scan with cuts of at least 5 millimeters is used to determine whether or not the patient has a unilateral adenoma versus bilateral adrenal hyperplasia as the cause of this hyperaldosteronism. When a solitary unilateral macroadenoma larger than 1 centimeter is found on CT scan in the presence of a normal contralateral adrenal, unilateral adrenalectomy is the treatment of choice. Depending on the preference of the surgeon, as well as the size of the lesion, laparoscopic or open surgical approaches may be used. In the case of bilateral abnormalities or microadenomas, adrenal venous sampling to search for a lateralizing source of the increased aldosterone is warranted. If lateralization is apparent, then surgery is indicated. If no lateralization is found, then spironolactone, a potassium-sparing diuretic, and followup is the treatment of choice.

The present patient had a PAC/PRA greater than 20. Because of this highly suspicious value, suggestive of hyperaldosteronism, she was evaluated further for Conn's syndrome. Following the implementation of a high-sodium diet for 3 days, 24-hour urine sodium and aldosterone levels were obtained. These values were indicative of primary hyperaldosteronism. Next, a spiral CT scan with 5-millimeter cuts through the adrenal gland was obtained. It demonstrated a 3-centimeter, solitary, unilateral left adrenal mass. A left adrenalectomy was performed. The patient tolerated the procedure well. Postoperatively, her hypertension and hypokalemia both resolved.

Clinical Pearls

1. Conn's syndrome is primary hyperaldosteronism causing hypertension, hypokalemia, hypernatremia, and metabolic alkalosis.

2. High aldosterone levels in the presence of sodium loading is pathognomonic of Conn's syndrome.

REFERENCES

1. Cook DM: Adrenal mass. Endocrinol Metab Clin North Am 26(4):829–852, 1997.
2. Vaughn ED Jr: Diagnosis of surgical adrenal disorders. AUA Update Series, Lesson 39, Vol XVI:306–311, 1997.
3. Young WF Jr: Pheochromocytoma and primary aldosteronism: Diagnostic approaches. Endocrinol Metab Clin North Am 26(4):801–827, 1997.

PATIENT 45

A newborn with ambiguous genitalia

A newborn child is transferred to the neonatal intensive care unit with a diagnosis of dehydration and failure to thrive. The child was born at 38 weeks of gestation to a healthy 22-year-old woman via normal, spontaneous, vaginal delivery. There were no complications during the pregnancy, and prenatal care was good. The child fed well initially, but soon began to feed poorly, vomit, and become lethargic.

Physical Examination: General: lethargic appearance; weak cry. Heart rate 190, blood pressure 40, respirations 25. Abdomen: soft, no masses palpable. Genitalia: enlarged phallus with significant chordee and a hypospadic opening; rugated scrotum with bilaterally nonpalpable testicles.

Laboratory Findings: Sodium 125 mEq/L, potassium 6.1 mEq/L, bicarbonate 19 mEq/L.

Questions: What is the most likely diagnosis? How should it be pursued?

Diagnosis: Ambiguous genitalia secondary to 21-hydroxylase deficiency

Discussion: Though ambiguous genitalia is an infrequent occurrence, it nonetheless comprises an extremely important group of medical disorders. In these emotionally sensitive cases it is critical that the precise etiology be delineated immediately so that any urgent metabolic abnormality can be treated quickly and safely, and the appropriate sex of rearing can be identified. Investigation of these disorders is best handled by a multidisciplinary team of physicians, including a urologist, pediatrician, geneticist, endocrinologist, and psychiatrist.

A cursory knowledge of normal sexual differentiation is helpful in understanding intersex abnormalities. Up until 6 weeks of age, the internal and external genitalia of the fetus is of an undifferentiated sex. Internally there is an indifferent gonad and both the mullerian and wolffian ducts, which become the female and male internal ducts, respectively. The external genitalia is represented by the genital tubercle, the urethral folds, and the labioscrotal folds.

The sex chromosomes direct the indifferent gonad to develop along male or female lines. The Y chromosome holds a testis-determining factor that causes the bipotential, undifferentiated gonad to develop into a testis. In the absence of the testis-determining factor, the bipotential gonad develops into an ovary. By the eighth week of development, the testis begins to secrete two hormones that help shape the internal and external duct system. Testosterone, produced by the Leydig cells, stimulates the wolffian duct to form the epididymis, vas deferens, and seminal vesicle. Mullerian inhibiting factor, produced by Sertoli cells, causes the regression of the mullerian duct system. At this early stage of development these hormones reach their targets by local diffusion and thus only affect the duct system ipsilateral to the gonad.

The concentration of testosterone reaches a maximum at 12 weeks, by which time the external genitals are developed in full. Testosterone is converted by 5-α-reductase to dihydrotestosterone. This leads to the formation of the glans (genital tubercle), anterior urethra (urethral folds), scrotum (genital swellings), and prostate (urogenital sinus) by the twelfth week. The penis, though perfectly formed at this stage, remains small until the third trimester.

The development of the female genitalia occurs mostly by an autonomous process. In the absence of testosterone and mullerian inhibiting factor, the mullerian ducts persist as the fallopian tubes, uterus, cervix, and upper vagina. The wolffian duct system regresses by the ninth week. In the absence of dihydrotestosterone, the clitoris (genital tubercle),

labia minora (urethral folds), labia majora (genital swellings), and lower vagina (urogenital sinus) develop.

The male embryo contains vestiges of the mullerian duct system in the form of the prostatic utricle and appendix testis. The female embryo contains vestiges of the wolffian duct system in the form of the epo-ophoron and Gartner's duct.

Intersex abnormalities generally are the result of abnormal fetal hormonal exposure. This abnormal exposure may be due to faulty chromosomal expression or coding, gonadal failure, target organ insensitivity, or overproduction of hormones from the fetus' adrenal or the mother's adrenal gland.

The criteria for investigation of potential intersex disorders are arbitrary. The incidence of an identifiable form of intersexuality increases as the severity of the degree of hypospadias or incomplete descent of a gonad increases.

Physical Appearances That Warrant Investigation

Male Phenotype	Intermediate	Female Phenotype
Bilateral impalpable testes	Ambiguous genitalia	Clitoral hypertrophy
Perineal hypospadias		Gonad in hernia sac
Unilateral undescended testis with hypospadias		Inseparably fused labia

From Aaronson IA: Sexual differentiation and intersexuality. In Kelalis PP, King LR, Belman AB (eds): Clinical Pediatric Urology, 3rd ed. Philadelphia, WB Saunders Co., 1992, pp 977–1014; with permission.

Despite comprehensive diagnostic criteria, some intersex cases only come to light in adolescence because of amenorrhea, inappropriate breast development, virilization, or onset of cyclical hematuria.

The investigation of an intersex patient is difficult to discuss with the new parents. It is important to initially offer a simple explanation, such as "Nature did not complete the differentiation of the genitalia, and further tests are needed to determine if the baby is a boy or a girl." At this point it is better to use the word baby, rather than he or she.

Once a definitive diagnosis has been established, an appropriate sex of rearing is agreed upon in a dialogue between the intersex team and the parents. The exact nature of the disorder and its long- and short-term implications are explained to the parents. With this information they are able to help the intersex team in identifying the sex of rearing.

Any clinical evaluation always starts with a history and physical examination. Find out whether any family members have had genital abnormalities, abnormal pubertal course, death in early infancy, or family history of infertility. Inquire about medications taken during pregnancy or hormonal usage. Physical examination is noteworthy for the presence or absence of testis and state of the external genitalia. Unequivocally, if one testis is palpable, then the patient is not a female pseudohermaphrodite. Size of the phallus and position of the meatus should be noted. Perform a rectal exam with a well lubricated finger to feel for a uterus. Look for abnormal skin pigmentation secondary to a high ACTH level, which suggests congenital adrenal hyperplasia.

Laboratory evaluation should include karyotyping to determine the exact chromosomal makeup of the patient. A biochemical evaluation pinpoints the metabolic defect that occurs in congenital adrenal hyperplasia—easily the most common cause of intersex abnormalities. Serum electrolytes must be evaluated for potentially lethal abnormalities. Serum and urine tests for various byproducts of the cortisol synthesis pathway can pinpoint the exact metabolic abnormality.

A genitogram should be carried out in all intersex cases. In children with congenital adrenal hyperplasia, the purpose of the study is to identify the level at which the vagina opens into the urogenital sinus with reference to the pelvic floor, to prepare for vaginoplasty. In other cases, its value is in its ability to identify the impression or outline of various internal organs. Other radiographic evaluation such as ultrasound can be used to determine the presence or absence of various intra-abdominal organs. However, ultrasound does not provide definitive answers.

In cases in which biochemical markers cannot be used to make a diagnosis, gonadal histology is important in establishing the cause of intersexuality. Palpable gonads are best exposed through an inguinal approach; impalpable ones via laparoscopy or laparotomy. Once the gonad has been found, a search for perigonadal structures should be made. A thin wedge biopsy may be excised, and a true pathological diagnosis can be formed.

An exhaustive review of all the causes of intersex abnormalities is impossible here. Here are the most common presentations and causes:

• **Male pseudohermaphroditism** is characterized by the presence of two normal testes. Genotypically, the patient is 46XY. Defective androgen production or sensitivity causes feminization or incomplete virilization of the external genitalia.

• **True hermaphroditism** is the least common of all intersex disorders. It is identified by the presence of both ovarian and testicular tissue (even the combined ovotestis) in the same patient. It has a variable genotypic presentation characterized by combinations of 46XX/46XY, 47XXX/46XY, or pure 46XX or 46XY. The clinical appearance varies widely, but most patients tend to be masculinized with large phalluses with chordee and a single urogenital sinus opening into a hypospadic position. The internal genitalia conform to the sex of the ipsilateral gonad.

• **Dysgenetic gonads** is another category of intersex disorders. The hallmark of these disorders is the disordered development of the gonads. Often the gonads are replaced by fibrous streaks. External genitalia and genetic makeup is variable, covering a full spectrum of presentations: from pure gonadal dysgenesis (e.g., Turner's syndrome, in which both ovaries are represented by fibrous streaks), to mixed gonadal dysgenesis (the most common of these disorders, with one gonad a fibrous streak and the other a testicle) all the way to testicular dysgenesis (in which the testes are purely dysplastic).

• **Female pseudohermaphroditism** is the most common cause of ambiguous genitalia. It is characterized by gonadal tissue represented by ovaries. The chromosomal analysis shows 46XX. Overexposure to androgens in utero causes severe masculinization of the external genitalia. **Congenital adrenal hyperplasia** is its most common cause, with 21-hydroxylase deficiency the most common form (accounts for 90% of the cases of congenital adrenal hyperplasia). These children show marked enlargement of the phallus, which excretes urine through a single urogenital sinus opening and is tethered by chordee. The labial folds are pigmented and rugaeted (appearing like a scrotum) due to excess ACTH. Many of these infants experience salt-wasting due to reduced aldosterone production, and the salt-wasting may cause a low plasma sodium and high renin and potassium levels. Death may occur in the neonatal period if the ensuing electrolyte abnormalities are unrecognized and untreated. Dehydration secondary to vomiting can lead to circulatory collapse. Internally, these children have female genital duct structures. Their ovaries may become polycystic.

Physicians need to be aware of the possibility of congenital adrenal hyperplasia as the cause of ambiguous genitalia in the newborn because of the possibility of **circulatory collapse**. Plasma electrolytes and blood pressure should be watched carefully. Plasma should be analyzed for elevated metabolites of cortisol synthesis, namely 17-hydroxyprogesterone and androstenedione. Hemodynamic support should be given to the infant as needed until the diagnosis is made and treatment with cortisol can begin. In those patients with the more severe salt-wasting variant, fluorocortisone is needed to bring plasma renin to normal levels. Most children outgrow the salt loss by the time they are 6 or 7 years old.

11-β-hydroxylase deficiency is the cause of 10% of the cases of congenital adrenal hyperplasia. It, too, causes buildup of 17-hydroxyprogesterone, but also causes buildup of deoxycorticosterone, resulting in salt retention. These children become hypertensive as they get older, and exhibit hypokalemia, acidosis, and normonatremia. Diagnosis is made by elevated serum 17-hydroxyprogesterone and 11-deoxycortisol.

Once a definitive diagnosis has been made in cases of ambiguous genitalia, the issue of sex assignment is of paramount importance. The entire intersex team, along with the parents, must make difficult, emotionally charged decisions. Criteria for determining the sex of rearing include age the child presents, ultimate fertility potential, anatomic considerations for reconstruction, need for future endocrine supplementation, potential for malignant change in the gonads, and genotypic makeup. Once a decision has been made, the need for and timing of surgery must be considered. Ultimately, these children can lead normal, productive lives.

The present patient was given immediate hemodynamic support. Fluid and electrolyte abnormalities were corrected. Plasma analysis demonstrated elevated 17-hydroxyprogesterone and androstenedione consistent with 21-hydroxylase deficiency. This child currently is undergoing radiographic and chromosomal analysis to better delineate the cause of the ambiguous genitalia, determine sex of rearing, and help plan for future treatment.

Clinical Pearls

1. Gonads are initially bipotential in all fetuses. If a Y chromosome is present, testis-determining factor is produced, and the gonad becomes a testis. In the absence of testis-determining factor, ovaries form.

2. Hypospadias coupled with impalpable testicles indicates an intersex abnormality, until proven otherwise.

3. Intersex abnormalities should be approached by a multidisciplinary team including a urologist, endocrinologist, pediatrician, geneticist, and psychiatrist.

4. The specific metabolic abnormality must be identified quickly to help treat any life-threatening problem.

5. Ambiguous genitalia can be categorized into four general areas: female pseudohermaphroditism, male pseudohermaphroditism, true hermaphroditism, and mixed gonadal dysgenesis.

6. Congenital adrenal hyperplasia is the most common cause of intersex abnormalities. 21-hydroxylase deficiency is the most common enzyme deficiency.

REFERENCES
1. Aaronson IA: Sexual differentiation and intersexuality. In Kelalis PP, King LR, Belman AB (eds): Clinical Pediatric Urology, 3rd ed. Philadelphia, WB Saunders Co., 1992, pp 977–1014.
2. Izquierdo G, Glassberg KI: Gender assignment and gender identity in patients with ambiguous genitalia. Urology 42(3):232–241, 1993.
3. Pang S: Congenital adrenal hyperplasia. Endocrinol Metab Clin North Am 26(4):853–858, 1997.

PATIENT 46

A 7-month-old boy with bilateral undescended testes

A 7-month-old boy has been referred by his pediatrician for further evaluation. The boy's mother states that he was noted to have bilateral undescended testes around the time of his birth. The patient was born at 38 weeks gestation and was of normal height and weight. He went home 2 days after his birth and has remained healthy since that time. The child takes no medication and has no known drug allergies.

Physical Examination: General: happy; appropriate appearance; in 60th percentile for height and weight. Cardiac: regular rate and rhythm, no murmur or rub. Chest: clear to auscultation bilaterally. Abdomen: soft, no masses. Genitalia: both testes palpable in inguinal canal, scrotum appropriately rugaeted, normal phallus. Back: no dimpling or other abnormality.

Laboratory Findings: None.

Question: If the testes had not been palpable in the inguinal canal, what physical exam clues would suggest that at least one testis is present?

Answer: A normal phallus and rugaeted scrotum suggest that at least one testicle is functioning and producing testosterone.

Discussion: An undescended testis is a testicle known to exist that did not migrate fully to rest in the scrotum. The term cryptorchidism frequently is used interchangeably with the term undescended testis, but the former more accurately describes a hidden testis that is not palpable. The incidence of undescended testes in newborn boys is 3–5%, with 15% being bilateral. This rate increases in certain situations, such as low birth weight, prematurity, and twinning. Boys with undescended testis are at higher risk for both infertility and testicular carcinoma. Recently, there has been a trend to operate earlier in the hope of improving long-term testicular function. Additionally, the use of laparoscopy has advanced both the diagnosis and treatment of the nonpalpable testis.

Testis development is an early embryologic event, while testis descent occurs in the third trimester. By the sixth week, primordial germ cells have migrated into the genital ridge on the ventromedial side of the mesonephros to form a bipotential gonad. Under influence of the SRY gene on the Y-chromosome, the gonad undergoes differentiation into a testis. By the ninth week, both Sertoli and Leydig cells have developed; these cells produce mullerian inhibiting factor and testosterone, respectively. The body of the epididymis and the vas deferens develop from the mesonephric tubules and wolffian duct structures. Additionally, by the ninth week the inferior attachment, termed the gubernaculum testis, is present.

Physical descent of the testes does not occur until after 28 weeks of gestation; however, there is some evidence that the testicle may be abnormal before the physical descent actually occurs. There are many proposed theories to explain testis descent, including gubernacular traction, hormonal influences, epididymal factors, and differential somatic growth. Some authors suggest that undescended testes result from an abnormality in the hypothalamic-pituitary-gonadal axis. This hypothesis is supported by the fact that children with CNS abnormalities have a high rate of bilateral undescended testes. Additionally, the normal postnatal surge in gonadotropins is blunted or absent in children with undescended testes, resulting in further testicular histologic abnormalities and possible future infertility.

An undescended testicle is at much greater risk of developing **testicular cancer** than a normal testicle. The risk of testicular cancer developing in a patient with an undescended testis is approximately 8 times higher than in the general population. Surgical placement of the testicle into the scrotum does not reduce the probability of developing cancer. However, it does aid in the surveillance of the testicle for tumor development. Another, weaker, association exists between an undescended testis and ipsilateral renal and ureteral abnormalities.

The classification of the undescended testicle is important for determining how to approach the testis for definitive therapy. The retractile testis is a testicle that has descended normally, but is retracted into the high scrotum by a vigorous cremasteric response. The retractile testicle is normal in size and histology. A history of a normal testicle at birth is suggestive. The true undescended testis, or cryptorchidism, may be located in the abdomen, in the high-annular (at the internal ring) position, the canalicular (the inguinal canal) position, the superficial inguinal position, or the high scrotal position. Additionally, the testis may occupy an ectopic position, such as the medial thigh or perineum.

The nonpalpable testicle requires special consideration. First, the patient must be examined thoroughly in a warm room in different postions, as at least 50% of patients referred to the pediatric urologist for a nonpalpable testis actually have a palpable testis. The physical exam is better than any radiologic imaging study in locating a testis. Upon surgical examination, 41% of abdominal testes were intracanalicular, 39% were in the intra-abdominal position, and 20% were missing or remnant tissue. Bilateral nonpalpable testes forces one to consider the possibility of hypogonadotropic hypogonadism, intersex, or the complete loss of functioning testicular tissue. The physical exam can aid by noting any signs of deficient **masculinization**, such as hypospadius or a hypoplastic scrotum, suggesting that indeed there is deficient testosterone production.

It is important to recognize that some testes that are undescended at birth naturally descend during the first 3 months of life. If the descent is not complete by that time, intervention is required. Treatment of an undescended testis ideally should occur around 1–2 years of age. Some recent data suggests that testicular function is better with early intervention. The goal of therapy is to maximize testicular function and place the testicle in the scrotum.

Hormonal therapy includes luteinizing hormone-releasing hormone (LHRH) and human chorionic gonadotropin (hCG), which can be given alone or in combination. Hormonal therapy is given, for a 2- to 3-week period after 6 months of age, for several reasons. First, some testes descend into the scrotum with hormonal therapy alone. Second, hormonal therapy has a maturing effect on the testicle, which improves its blood supply, making the testicle better able to withstand the Fowler-Stevens procedure (described at right). Third, some data suggests that early hormonal therapy improves later fertility.

Surgical treatment is employed in the majority of patients with undescended testes. For the testicle that is palpable, most surgeons would opt for an inguinal incision to identify the testicle and bring it into the scrotum. For testes that are not palpable, a laparoscopic approach can be used to identify either the testicle or the blind-ending gonadal vessels of an absent testicle. The laparoscope can then be used to assist in bringing the testicle into the scrotum. Occasionally, special procedures are used to bring a high testicle into the scrotum. One of these approaches is known as the Fowler-Stevens procedure, in which the gonadal vessels are cut, and the testicle is brought down with the vas deferens and the deferential blood supply. In adults, most surgeons would opt for orchiectomy on an undescended testis, assuming a normally functioning contralateral testis, due to the risk of cancer.

The present patient underwent a course of LHRH for three weeks. Re-examination at the end of that period revealed that both testicles remained in the inguinal canal. At 1 year of age the boy underwent a bilateral orchidopexy to bring both of his testicles into his scrotum. He tolerated the procedure well and can be expected to develop normally. Monthly testicular self-exams should be started early in the adolescent period.

Clinical Pearls

1. Many undescended testes descend during the first 3 months of life.
2. Physical exam is the most sensitive modality for locating an undescended testis.
3. Undescended testes have a relative risk for testicular cancer approximately eight-fold that of normal testes; this is not altered by bringing the testicle into the scrotum.
4. Early surgical intervention and hormonal therapy may improve later testicular function.

REFERENCES
1. Rozanski TA, Bloom DA: The undescended testis: Theory and management. Urol Clin North Am 22:107–117, 1995.
2. Gillenwater JY, Grayhack JT, Howards SS, Duckett JW (eds): Adult and Pediatric Urology. St. Louis, Mosby-Year Book, Inc., 1996.
3. Cortes D: Cryptorchidism—aspects of pathogenesis, histology and treatment. Scand J Urol Nephrol 196:1–54, 1998.

PATIENT 47

A 22-year-old man with gross hematuria following a motorcycle accident

A 22-year-old man is brought to the trauma bay in the emergency department following a motorcycle accident. The paramedic from the scene reports that the man was driving approximately 30 miles per hour when he was hit at a low velocity from the side by an automobile. The man was thrown from his motorcycle and struck a retaining wall with his pelvis and right flank. The patient denies any significant past medical history and is not taking any medications. He reports never losing consciousness and complains now of right leg, right flank, and pelvic pain.

Physical Examination: **Primary survey.** General: anxious, but talking to staff; clothes torn on right side; several obvious minor lacerations and contusions on right side; no respiratory difficulty. Temperature 36.6°, respirations 20, pulse 120, blood pressure 120/82. Glasgow coma score: 15/15. **Secondary survey.** Cardiac: no longer tachycardic, no murmur or rub. Chest: clear to auscultation bilaterally. Abdomen: soft, nontender, no rebound tenderness. Flanks: right ecchymosis, right tender to palpation. Pelvis: unstable, right upper thigh ecchymosis. Genitalia: blood at the urethral meatus, blood-stained urine noted in underpants. Rectal: difficult to palpate prostate. Extremities: normal peripheral pulses, no gross deformity.

Laboratory Findings: Initial chest, pelvis, and cervical spine x-rays: right pubic ramus fracture, right 12th rib fracture, normal cervical spine. Other data not available yet.

Questions: What is the diagnosis? What two radiographic studies should be obtained to confirm this diagnosis?

Answer: Posterior urethral injury. A high-dose intravenous pyelogram and a retrograde urethrogram should be obtained.

Discussion: Trauma is the leading cause of death in people aged 1 to 44 years. This group obviously represents people with many years of productive life ahead of them. In 1976, an orthopedic surgeon and his children were injured when his private plane crashed; his wife was killed instantly. The surgeon recognized that the care his family received was inadequate, and from his experience was born a standardized, thorough approach to the evaluation and treatment of the trauma patient. This approach is taught in the Advanced Trauma Life Support course. All of the necessary information is obtained in less than 10 minutes. The urethral injury is focused on in this discussion. However, it is important to recognize that this patient was at high risk for a renal injury in addition to his urethral injury.

The male urethra comprises four regions: the prostatic, membranous, bulbous, and penile. They are divided into the posterior (prostatic and membranous) urethra and the anterior (bulbous and penile) urethra. Due to the fact that the prostatic urethra is attached to the bony pelvis via the puboprostatic ligaments, and the membranous urethra is held by the urogenital diaphragm, shearing forces place the male urethra at high risk of injury from pelvic trauma. This is in contrast to the female urethra, which seldom is injured secondary to traumatic pelvic injuries.

The majority of urethral injuries are to the posterior urethra, of which 90% are caused by motor vehicle accidents. The anterior urethra also is subject to traumatic injury, but anterior urethra injuries usually are a result of trauma to the perineum, as in a straddle injury. Penetrating trauma, such as knife and gunshot wounds, may damage the urethra as well; however, these injuries are much less common. Posterior urethral injuries are classified into three categories: Type I injuries occur when the prostatic attachments to the urogenital diaphragm are disrupted, resulting in a hematoma that compresses the prostatomembranous urethra; there is no actual urethral disruption. Type II occur when the prostatomembranous urethra is disrupted at the apex of the prostate. Type III injuries are most common and are the same as type II with the addition of injury to the urogenital diaphragm and the bulbous urethra.

The diagnosis of a urethral injury should be suspected in any man who has suffered trauma to the perineum or who has a pelvic fracture. The patient may complain that he has the urge to void but is unable, or that when voiding he notes no urine from the penis. Signs that indicate urethral trauma include blood at the meatus and perineal, penile, or scrotal hematoma. Additionally, a high-riding prostate or a boggy prostatic fossa may be present. The prostate findings are attributed to loss of the prostatic attachments to the urogenital diaphragm or to a hematoma in the prostatic fossa.

If suspicion of a urethral injury exists, a retrograde urethrogram is performed to make the diagnosis. A 14 French Foley catheter is inserted 2–3 centimeters from the fossa navicularis. The Foley catheter balloon is then filled with 1–2 cubic centimeters of water just to hold the catheter in place. Approximately 25 cubic centimeters of dilute contrast is injected through the Foley catheter with the patient in an oblique position, and several x-rays are obtained. Ideally, this study should be performed under fluoroscopic monitoring. If the study reveals that the urethra is normal, then the Foley catheter balloon can be deflated and reinserted, or exchanged for a larger catheter if necessary. *Under no circumstances should a Foley catheter be placed into the bladder before a retrograde urethrogram is performed if there is suspicion of urethral injury.* A partial urethral tear can be converted to a more serious, complete disruption by the careless passing of a Foley catheter.

Appropriate management of posterior urethral injury is required to minimize long-term complications resulting from injury and attempted repair. Type I injuries require only the placement of a Foley catheter for several days as the tissue edema and hematoma resolve. Type II and Type III injuries are divided into partial or complete tear categories. **Partial urethral tears**, if they are minimal, may be managed by the careful passage of a Foley catheter. If any resistance is met, this approach should be aborted, and a suprapubic tube should be placed for 14–21 days. After that period, the injury should be re-evaluated with a voiding cystourethrogram (VCUG). **Complete urethral tears** can be handled either with immediate or delayed surgical repair. In recent years, delayed surgical repair has become the preferred treatment option for the majority of patients. Studies have demonstrated that there are lower rates of impotence, incontinence, and stricture recurrence with delayed repair. The indications in which immediate repair might still be considered are the following: the patient is stable and has a severe disruption with a "pie-in-the-sky bladder," or the patient is stable but requires pelvic exploration for other, associated injuries. However, for most patients the most appropriate management is placement of a suprapubic catheter, which remains in place for 6 months while the pelvis heals. Then a VCUG and retrograde urethrogram are performed, and the most appropriate surgical repair is planned. An intravenous pyelogram is done to exclude the presence of injuries to the upper tract.

Anterior urethral injuries are managed by immediate Foley catheter placement, and the catheter is left in place for several days. The exception to this management occurs if there is complete disruption with no filling of the bladder on retrograde urethrogram. In this case, a suprapubic catheter is placed and repair delayed.

In the present patient, a high-dose IVP was normal. A retrograde urethrogram revealed contrast extravasation at the posterior urethra, confirming the diagnosis. He underwent the immediate placement of a suprapubic tube in the emergency department. The suprapubic tube remained in place with monthly catheter changes for 6 months while the pelvis healed. After 6 months, the patient had a VCUG and retrograde urethrogram, both of which demonstrated a 1.5-centimeter membranous urethral stricture. The stricture was repaired with an open primary stricture incision and urethral reanastomosis shortly thereafter. The patient has experienced no further difficulties.

Clinical Pearls

1. Urethral injury should be suspected in any male who has sustained a pelvic fracture or perineal trauma.

2. Clinical signs and symptoms may include the following: blood at the meatus, a high-riding prostate, and ecchymosis of the penis, scrotum, or perineum.

3. Diagnosis of urethral injury is made by retrograde urethrogram.

4. A Foley catheter should never be inserted into a patient at high risk for urethral injury until that injury has been ruled out.

5. Patients have a lower long-term complication rate with delayed repair. Therefore, the majority of these patients should be treated with immediate suprapubic tube placement.

REFERENCES

1. Lim PH, Chung HC: Initial management of acute urethral injuries. Br J Urol 64:165, 1989.
2. American College of Surgeons Committee on Trauma: Advanced Trauma Life Support. Chicago, American College of Surgeons, 1993.
3. Gillenwater JY, Grayhack JT, Howards SS, Duckett JW (eds): Adult and Pediatric Urology, 3rd ed. St. Louis, Mosby-Year Book, Inc., 1996.

PATIENT 48

A 21-year-old woman with a gunshot wound to the abdomen and gross hematuria

A 21-year-old woman arrives in the trauma bay of the emergency department following a gunshot wound to the right mid abdomen. The paramedic from the scene reports that the woman was accidentally shot once in the abdomen with a small-caliber handgun that was kept in her home. The patient told the paramedic that she has no past medical history, is not taking any medications, and has no known allergies.

Physical Examination: **Primary survey.** General: alert; complaining of abdominal pain; pale; blood on shirt over abdomen. Temperature: 36.4°, pulse 130, blood pressure 90/60, respirations 30. Glasgow coma score: 13/15. **Secondary survey.** blood pressure 100/74; pulse 110. Cardiac: tachycardic, no rub or murmur. Chest: clear to auscultation bilaterally. Abdomen: soft, diffuse tenderness greater on the right; positive rebound tenderness; small entrance wound over right mid abdomen. Extremities: normal peripheral pulses. Back: exit wound on right side; right flank ecchymosis. Rectum: negative.

Laboratory Findings: Foley catheter: 150 cubic centimeters bloody urine. Chest x-ray: negative. Other data not available yet.

Question: What diagnostic study specific to the genitourinary system should be performed while the patient is being further evaluated and treated?

Answer: A high-dose intravenous pyelogram

Discussion: The kidney is the most frequently injured genitourinary organ in both blunt and penetrating trauma. Approximately 8–10% of blunt and penetrating trauma involves the kidneys. Blunt trauma is more common than penetrating trauma; therefore, most renal injuries are the result of blunt trauma. However, approximately 20% of renal injuries in large urban centers occur as a result of penetrating trauma. Gunshot wounds comprise the majority of penetrating traumatic injuries, but stab wounds and impalement also are possible causes.

The severity of renal injury is classified into five categories. Grade I is a renal contusion or subcapsular hematoma. Grade II is a renal cortical laceration less than 1 centimeter deep. Grade III is a laceration greater than 1 centimeter deep that may involve the medulla, but does not involve the collecting system. Grade IV injuries are lacerations that involve the cortex, the medulla, and the collecting system, or injuries to the renal artery or vein with a contained hematoma. Grade V injuries include a shattered kidney or avulsion of the renal artery or vein.

The overwhelming majority of patients with a renal injury have gross or microscopic hematuria (more than 5–10 RBC/hpf). However, this is not always the case, particularly if traumatic renal artery occlusion exists. Therefore, a high index of suspicion should always exist for the possibility of renal injury. Interestingly, the degree of hematuria is not a good predictor of the seriousness of injury. Some additional signs and symptoms of a renal injury in a patient with blunt abdominal trauma are: abdominal/flank tenderness, flank ecchymosis, and lower rib fracture. Penetrating renal injuries always should be suspected in a patient who has sustained a gunshot wound to the abdomen.

The diagnosis of a renal injury usually is made by either high-dose intravenous pyelogram (IVP) or CT scan. Indications for imaging in blunt trauma are (1) gross hematuria or (2) microscopic hematuria and shock (blood pressure less than 90 mmHg). In penetrating trauma, all patients inciting suspicion of kidney injury or with any degree of hematuria (more than 5 RBC/hpf) should be studied. The decision on whether to image using CT scan or IVP depends on the expected management of the patient. If the patient has other indications for a CT scan or there are no immediate plans to take the patient to the operating room for exploration, a CT scan is preferred because much more information is attained. A high-dose of IVP is simple and fast. It should be preceded by a kidneys, ureter, and bladder (KUB) x-ray examination. After an injection of IV contrast at a dose of 2 cubic centimeters per kilogram, x-rays in the KUB position are taken, preferably with nephrotomograms.

Indications for operative intervention vary slightly from institution to institution, but some helpful guidelines exist. Absolute indications for operative intervention include either an expanding or pulsatile hematoma. Relative indications include urine extravasation, any type of vascular injury, and nonviable parenchyma, particularly if 20% or more of renal parenchyma is involved. Penetrating renal injuries usually are associated with other abdominal injuries; therefore, the management of this injury type is surgical exploration. However, the majority of blunt renal trauma is a Grade I contusion not requiring surgical intervention. The decision to operate on any patient who does not fall easily into the operative or conservative management categories should be with the goal of minimizing complications. For example, give careful consideration to the operative management of a patient with a Grade IV injury who has a small hematoma, a small urinoma, and a nonviable lower pole, because there is an expected high incidence of complications such as infection, persistent extravasation, and delayed bleeding.

The management of renal injury requires a high index of suspicion, knowledge of what factors put the patient at high risk for renal injury, and the ability to choose the most appropriate diagnostic study. Additionally, the ability to analyze the data to make an operative versus conservative management decision based on the desire to minimize morbidity and mortality is required.

The present patient was in shock when she first arrived in the trauma room. Rapid resuscitation and diagnosis were of the utmost importance. Her shock was temporarily reversed, and right renal injury was diagnosed based on the nature of the injury and the presence of hematuria. A high-dose IVP was done, rather than a CT scan, because the patient presented in shock and will have to undergo surgical exploration. If the patient had not responded to resuscitation, she would have been taken to the operating room immediately with all further evaluation suspended. A severe Grade IV or Grade V injury was suggested by the results of the high-dose IVP.

The patient clearly met the indications for operative intervention and was taken to the operating room. Due to the high likelihood of other injuries, a midline incision was used to expose the viscera and the kidney. A renal artery injury was discovered, and control of the vascular structures was obtained. The patient remained stable intraoperatively; therefore, a careful arterial repair was undertaken successfully.

Clinical Pearls

1. Renal injury should be suspected in a blunt trauma patient who has gross hematuria or has microscopic hematuria associated with shock. Any patient with penetrating trauma and microscopic (> 5 RBC/hpf) or gross hematuria should be suspected of having underlying renal injury.

2. High-dose IVP can be performed quickly and easily in the trauma bay to diagnose most significant renal injuries.

3. The majority of blunt, traumatic renal injury is Grade I, requiring no operative intervention. The majority of penetrating trauma requires operative intervention.

REFERENCES

1. McAninch JW: Renal trauma. In Resnick MI (ed): Current Trends in Urology. Vol 3. Baltimore, Williams & Wilkins, 1985.
2. American College of Surgeons Committee on Trauma: Advanced Trauma Life Support. Chicago, American College of Surgeons, 1993.
3. Gillenwater JY, Grayhack JT, Howards SS, Duckett JW (eds): Adult and Pediatric Urology, 3rd ed. St. Louis, Mosby-Year Book, Inc., 1996.

PATIENT 49

A 44-year-old spinal cord–injured patient with foul-smelling urine

A 44-year-old man with a T10 complete spinal cord lesion is admitted to the hospital with fevers to 39.1°C, chills, and foul-smelling urine. He has been a spinal cord patient for 7 years and manages his urine output with a condom catheter. He has one or two febrile urinary tract infections (UTI) a year. He is followed by a family physician. Prior radiographs and urodynamic studies are not available. The patient is not taking any medications.

Physical Examination: Temperature 39.1°; pulse 118; respirations 28; blood pressure 90/50. Chest: clear. Cardiac: normal heart tones, no murmurs. Abdomen: soft, nontender; no pressure ulcers. Genitalia: circumcised, normal.

Laboratory Findings: WBC 24,000/μl, hemoglobin 12 mg/dl. Electrolytes, BUN, creatinine: normal. Urinalysis via straight catheter: pH 6, nitrite positive, LE positive, 50–100 RBC/hpf, 100 WBC/hpf, 3+ bacteria. Urine culture: pending. Right renal ultrasound: normal. Left renal ultrasound: see figure.

Question: How are the fever, urine pH, microscopic findings on urinalysis, and ultrasound findings significant?

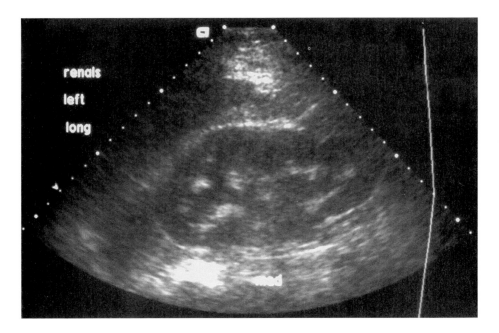

Diagnosis: Febrile urinary tract infection and a neurogenic bladder with incomplete emptying

Discussion: Spinal cord–injured (SCI) patients represent one of the most challenging groups in urologic care. These patients require a logical and rational approach to their long-term management, as urologic complications are perhaps the most common causes of morbidity and mortality. Improvements in knowledge of urodynamic dysfunction, its treatment, and the management of complications are largely responsible for the improved survival of SCI patients.

Normal bladders store urine at low pressures. They empty via coordinated detrusor muscle contraction, with bladder neck and sphincter relaxation. Storage of urine under low pressures is related to sympathetic input from T10–12 to the bladder body and neck and compliant viscoelastic properties of the bladder. Detrusor contraction is integrated in the parasympathetic sacral reflex center at S2–4. Volitional control of voiding resides in the cerebral cortex. Under normal conditions, sensory afferents in the detrusor sense fullness and relay the signal to the sacral center. This signal is relayed along the dorsal columns of the spinal cord to the pontine micturition center, then onto the cerebral cortex. The cerebral cortex can suppress the reflex if not convenient to void. If voiding is desirable, impulses return via the spinal cord to T10–12 and S2–4 for a coordinated detrusor contraction and bladder neck and sphincter relaxation. In the absence of anatomic barriers to voiding, normal voiding occurs. SCI disrupts the pathways between S2–4 and the pons, with a fairly predictable outcome.

SCI produces a dyscoordination between detrusor contraction and bladder outlet opening. This is known as detrusor external sphincter dysynergia (DESD). All SCI patients have some degree of DESD, but whether or not the patients empty their bladder adequately at low detrusor pressures is the critical factor. Goals of management are to keep the patient free from leakage of urine while storing it at low pressures and enable emptying of the bladder on a routine, frequent schedule. Urodynamic evaluation, including cystometrograms, sphincter electromyelograms, and renal ultrasounds, dictates the best management plan. The plan usually involves intermittent self-catheterization (CIC), with anticholinergic, alpha blocker, or alpha adrenergic medication added as needed based on the clinical, radiographic, and urodynamic findings.

Urinary tract infections (UTIs) may be classified as either simple or complicated. A simple UTI occurs in a person with an entirely normal urinary tract, and if the UTI is treated appropriately, it resolves completely. SCI patients do not have normal urinary tracts, so, by definition, UTIs in SCI patients are complicated. The problem arises in differentiating infection from colonization. The majority of SCI patients are managed by either CIC or condom catheter. The remainder are managed by chronic indwelling catheters. CIC is associated with asymptomatic bacteriuria in 60% of patients, compared to 50% of patients with condom catheters. Patients with chronic indwelling catheters no doubt are at greatest risk for bacteriuria, with a 10% incidence per day and a 75–90% incidence at 60 days. These figures refer to asymptomatic "colonization," since patients on CIC have only 1.8 episodes of symptomatic UTI with fever and chills on average per year.

The critical issue involves distinguishing which patients are infected and which are not. In normal patients, UTIs typically are associated with irritative voiding symptoms and **fevers**, chills, or flank pain. SCI patients often do not have these symptoms. Complaints such as malaise, decreased appetite, fevers, vague back or belly discomfort, or leakage between self-catheterizations or around indwelling catheters may indicate the presence of a UTI. Other infections, such as pneumonia or osteomyelitis, should be ruled out. Eliciting information regarding prior infectious episodes, prior surgical procedures, medication history, and method of bladder drainage is important. Old radiograph and urodynamic studies should be obtained, if possible. Laboratory analyses should include CBC, serum electrolytes, BUN, creatinine, urine analysis, and urine culture.

Interpretation of the urine specimen is challenging. First, knowledge of how the specimen was collected is important to rule out contamination. Straight catheterized specimens are optimal. Second, urinalysis findings that define a UTI are debatable. A high percentage of these patients have bacteriuria and pyuria in the absence of clinical infection. Urinary nitrites, leukocyte esterase, and **pH** all have been used in an effort to define urinary infection. However, not all bacteria produce nitrites, and leukocyte esterase merely indicates the presence of white blood cells, so these tests are neither sensitive nor specific. A urine pH above 7.5, however, requires further scrutiny and culture to identify urea-splitting organisms, because they can produce infection stones. If found on culture, the organisms should be treated, and the urinary tract should be imaged for the presence of stones.

Pyuria has been used by some in an effort to distinguish infected from noninfected urine. In non-SCI patients with UTIs, pyuria is present approximately 98% of the time. Pyuria in SCI patients is variable and largely depends on the method of bladder drainage. Both CIC and indwelling catheters may be associated frequently with pyuria. Thus, the presence of pyuria has low positive predictive value for infection. Pyuria and bacteriuria should be interpreted amongst the constellation of available data and not relied upon as a single entity.

Imaging studies should be obtained at some point during the hospital course—the timing depends on the patient's condition—to look for hydronephrosis, stones, and fungus balls, and to examine general renal and bladder appearance. Options include ultrasound, CT scan, IVP, and plain abdominal x-rays. **Ultrasound** probably is the optimal initial study, since it is inexpensive, safe, and sensitive for most of the above findings. A finding of hydronephrosis should be interpreted with caution because it may represent chronic ectatic changes, not obstruction. The patient's clinical condition dictates conservative management versus intervention in the form of retrograde or percutaneous antegrade renal drainage. A radionucleotide renal scan can assess differential renal function and distinguish nonobstructive from obstructive pyelectasis.

Initial management should begin with a global assessment of the patient's condition, fluid resuscitation, placement of a urinary catheter, unless already in place, and broad-spectrum antimicrobial therapy. Ampicillin or pipiricillin with gentamicin should cover the vast majority of uropathogens, including *Escherichia coli*, Pseudomonas sp., Klebsiella, Seratia, Providencia, Proteus, and Enterococcus. Aztreonam or quinolones may substitute for gentamicin in the renally impaired patient. In the stable outpatient, a course of oral quinolones may be tried. These agents achieve excellent urinary concentrations with a good spectrum for uropathogens and have equivalent bioavailability in the oral and parenteral forms. Empiric therapy should be guided by hospital-specific susceptibility patterns; antimicrobials can be tailored appropriately once susceptibility tests return. Patients should recover quickly on appropriate therapy, though continued fever spikes for 2–3 days are common. Failure to improve after several days warrants repeat culturing, re-evaluation of antimicrobials, and repeat radiographic imaging.

The present patient was admitted to the hospital for intravenous antimicrobials due to his high fevers and leukocytosis. The lack of physical findings suggesting infection elsewhere, combined with the fevers, CBC, and urinary findings, were highly suggestive of a urinary source of infection. The urine pH of 6 was significant for indicating the absence of urea-splitting bacteria and the unlikelihood of infection stones. The patient underwent an ultrasound examination on admission, mostly because he had not had one in several years. (Since bladder function may change over time in SCI patients, these patients should be followed with yearly renal ultrasounds.) The ultrasound revealed hydronephrosis, the implications of which were unclear at that time. Since his clinical condition was improving, he was followed conservatively, and a Foley catheter was placed. Followup ultrasound several days later, with the Foley in place, was unchanged. The patient subsequently underwent a radionucleotide renal scan the following day, which demonstrated good excretion, i.e., no functional obstruction. The hydronephrosis thus was considered a chronic change—most likely due to chronic urodynamic changes in a neurogenic bladder. His condition continued improving and his urine culture grew more than 100,000 colony-forming units of pan-sensitive *E. coli*. The antimicrobials were tailored accordingly, and he was discharged home on oral trimethoprim-sulfa with a followup appointment for urodynamic studies and a re-evaluation of his bladder management regimen.

Clinical Pearls

1. The majority of patients with spinal cord injuries have bacteriuria, which may not represent symptomatic infection.

2. Treating asymptomatic bacteriuria selects for multidrug-resistant organisms and should be avoided.

3. No one indicator (symptom, sign, or laboratory value) accurately distinguishes infection from colonization.

4. Urine with a pH greater than 7.5 should be cultured to rule out the presence of urea-splitting organisms. The genitourinary tract should be imaged to rule out stones.

REFERENCES

1. Cardenas DD, Hooton TM: Urinary tract infection in persons with spinal cord injury. Arch Phys Med Rehabil 76:272–280, 1995.
2. Kreder KJ, Nygaard IE: Spine Update: Urologic management in patients with spinal cord injuries. Spine 21:128–132, 1996.
3. Watanabe T, Rivas DA, Chanellor MB: Urodynamics of spinal cord injury. Urol Clin North Am 23:459–469, 1996.
4. Bergman SB, Yarkony GM, Stiens SA: Spinal Cord Injury. 2. Medical Complications. Arch Phys Med Rehabil 78:53–58, 1997.

PATIENT 50

A 44-year-old woman with total urinary incontinence after a total abdominal hysterectomy

A 44-year-old woman complains of constant vaginal discharge 2 weeks after a total abdominal hysterectomy for the treatment of uterine fibroids. She is healthy otherwise and takes no medications.

Physical Examination: Afebrile; blood pressure 120/70; respirations 22. General: healthy appearance. Abdomen: well-healing lower midline transverse incision. Genitalia: malodorous, clear discharge with perineal skin masceration; perivulvar papular rash with satellite papules.

Laboratory Findings: Complete blood cell count: normal. Sequential Multiple Analysis-7: normal. Urinalysis: RBC 100/hpf, WBC 100/hpf, 3+ budding yeast. BUN 55 mg/dl, creatinine 10 mg/dl. Urine culture: positive for candidal infection.

Question: What is the significance of constant vaginal leakage after a hysterectomy?

Diagnosis: Vesicovaginal fistula

Discussion: Vesicovaginal fistula (VVF) is a rare but devastating condition of multiple etiologies. In the United States and other developed nations, it is primarily the result of one operation: the abdominal hysterectomy. The incidence of VVF in this operation is 1%, and approximately 50% of VVFs are due to abdominal hysterectomies. Other causes in this country include transvaginal surgery, retropubic surgery, laparoscopic surgery, pelvic infections, vaginal foreign bodies, pelvic malignancies, radiation injuries, and congenital anomalies. In developing nations VVFs are most commonly an obstetrical complication, secondary to prolonged or obstructed labor.

The hallmark of the VVF is vaginal leakage or total urinary incontinence days to weeks after a hysterectomy. Patients also may complain of abdominal pain, ileus, hematuria, irritative voiding symptoms, or excessive discharge from vaginal or abdominal wounds. History may reveal prior abdominal, pelvic, or transvaginal surgery. Risk factors include malignancy, endometriosis, pelvic infectious disorders, corticosteroid use, or prior pelvic irradiation. Radiation-induced fistulae may occur months to years after completion of treatment. In such patients, recurrent cancer should be excluded with biopsy.

Diagnosis of VVF is usually straightforward. The patient will have the appropriate history and risk factors, with physical exam revealing the stigmata of prior surgical procedures. Inspection of the perineum and vagina often shows macerated, inflamed skin, the rash of yeast infection, and a malodorous discharge. Chemical analyses of the discharge reveals a BUN and creatinine consistent with urinary values. Speculum exam may reveal the fistulous connection, if it is large. Cystoscopic signs include mucosal inflammation and granulation tissue. Urinary dye tests with intravaginal gauze have been described to assist in diagnosis. In these tests, methylene blue is placed in the bladder via a catheter, and a gauze pad is placed in the vagina, allowing staining of the vaginal gauze if a VVF is present. Staining the pad after the intravenous administration of methylene blue indicates an associated ureterovaginal fistula (UVF). UVF occurs 10–12% of the time in association with VVF and needs to be excluded.

Radiographic imaging should be performed to document the injury and to rule out an associated UVF. Intravenous pyelogram, retrograde pyelography, and voiding cystourethrography are useful. Cystoscopy and vaginoscopy aid in planning repair and can define the number of fistulae, their size, their relationship to the ureters, and associated or concurrent bladder and vaginal pathology.

Management of VVF classically entails a 3- to 6-month wait period in which conservative attempts are made to correct the disorder. The psychological ramifications of suffering months of total urinary incontinence; malodor; irritated, macerated skin; and vaginal and bladder infections complicate this approach. In addition, in uncomplicated VVF, i.e., not associated with radiation, success rates are equivalent to early versus delayed repairs. A waiting period is appropriate for radiation-induced fistulae, and there is evidence that hyperbaric oxygen therapy may promote healing.

The general approach to these patients depends on the size and number of the fistulae. For small fistulae (< 1 centimeter), an attempt at Foley drainage and anticholinergic medication has a 10–12% success rate for spontaneous closure. Additional conservative measures include de-epithelializing the tract with curettage or coagulation. When these measures are unsuccessful, or for large or multiple fistulae, open repair is indicated.

Options for open repair include transvaginal and abdominal procedures. In both, the same basic surgical principles apply. Tissue must be approximated free of tension and well vascularized, and necrotic and inflamed tissue must be debrided. In cases where tension-free repairs are not possible, vascularized flaps should be employed. The most commonly used abdominal and vaginal flaps are the omental flap and the Martius labial fat pad flap. The fistulous tract does not need to be excised, as long as the repair may be performed tension free, with healthy, viable tissue.

Abdominal and transvaginal repairs are equally effective. The method used often depends on the skill and preference of the surgeon, patient preferences, and the complexity of the required procedures. The majority of VVFs can be appropriately managed by the transvaginal route. Patients recover well and have minimal postoperative morbidity. Moreover, it allows for concurrent pelvic floor reconstruction and avoids re-entering the abdominal cavity in previously operated patients. The transvaginal route even can be used in previously radiated patients. Preoperative hyperbaric oxygen therapy may increase the likelihood of a successful outcome in these challenging cases.

Abdominal approaches provide optimal exposure in multiple VVFs, fistulae involving multiple organs, or associated UVFs requiring ureteral reimplantation. In cases of a single VVF with poor exposure transvaginally, the abdominal route is preferable.

Patients usually do very well postoperatively. Bladder spasm can be ameliorated with adequate drainage and anticholinergic medication. Most surgeons use both urethral and suprapubic vesical drainage. In complex repairs, the addition of externalized ureteral stenting may be useful. Broad-spectrum antimicrobials should be used until the catheters and stents have been removed, usually 2–3 weeks later. In an uncommon subset of patients with recalcitrant fistulae or those associated with recurrent malignancy, palliation may be achieved with urinary diversion.

This patient presented in a manner classic for a VVF. The associated rash is characteristic of candida infection, and the findings of urinary levels of BUN and creatinine suggest the diagnosis. A cystoscopy and a retrograde pyelogram revealed a single 1-centimeter fistula at the dome of the bladder, without an associated UVF. The patient initially elected conservative management—anticholinergic medication and Foley drainage—without resolution. She subsequently underwent a transvaginal repair and has since been without problems.

Clinical Pearls

1. Any woman with total incontinence or excessive vaginal discharge after a hysterectomy should be considered to have a vesicovaginal fistula.
2. An associated ureterovaginal fistula must be ruled out.
3. Only 10% of patients with VVF will heal with conservative measures.
4. In cases of prior radiation therapy for malignancy, recurrent cancer must be ruled out by biopsy.

REFERENCES
1. Mercer LJ, Margolis T: Vesicovaginal fistula. Obstetrical and Gynecological Survey 49:840–847, 1994.
2. McAninch JW (ed): Traumatic and Reconstructive Urology. Philadelphia, W.B. Saunders Company, 1996.
3. Rackley RR, Appell RA: Vesicovaginal fistula: Current approach. AUA Update Series 17, lesson 28, 162–167, 1998.

PATIENT 51

A 27-year-old man with a pelvic fracture after a motor vehicle accident

A 27-year-old man was involved in a high-speed (approximately 60 mph) motor vehicle collision. The car was severely damaged, with a bent steering wheel. At the scene, he is lethargic but arousable, with a blood pressure of 90. Intravenous access is established in the field, and he is brought into the emergency department where more extensive intravenous access is initiated. A Foley catheter is passed via his urethra, without meeting any resistance. There is no urine output.

Physical Examination: General: no external bleeding or angulation. **Primary survey.** Pulse: normal. Cardiac: tachycardia after 2 liters of rapidly infused Ringer's lactate solution; heart tones normal. Chest: clear lungs; equal breath sounds bilaterally; steering wheel–shaped ecchymosis. Abdomen: soft and diffusely tender; lower distension. Genitalia: absence of blood at meatus; normal testicles; prostate normal. Back: no cervical spine tenderness.

Laboratory Findings: Hemoglobin 11 mg/dl. Electrolytes, BUN, creatinine: normal. Blood alcohol content: 240 mg/dl. Radiographs: normal cervical spine; chest normal; pelvic film and cystogram obtained (see figures); no retrograde urethrogram performed.

Questions: Why was a retrograde urethrogram not performed? Why was a cystogram performed?

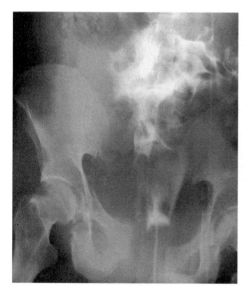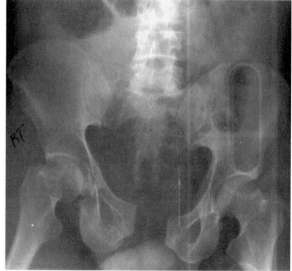

Diagnosis: Posterior urethral complete disruption with an intraperitoneal bladder rupture secondary to pelvic ring fracture

Discussion: Pelvic fractures represent life-threatening injuries and are associated with injuries to multiple organ systems. The force required to produce a pelvic ring disruption is considerable, which is why associated injuries are common. Thus, the urologist needs to be well versed in urologic sequelae to pelvic fracture. Genitourinary injuries, while rarely life threatening, can cause significant long-term disability, which may be minimized if appropriately managed initially.

The pelvis consists of a ring of bones and ligaments surrounding highly vascular organs. As a ring, isolated fracture to one ring segment is impossible. Pelvic structures such as bladder neck, prostate, urethra, and vagina are anchored at various points to the pelvic ring. The blood supply comes mainly from anterior and posterior divisions of the hypogastric artery, and the nerve supply arises from the sacral and pelvis plexuses. It is not difficult to imagine that a force great enough to fracture the pelvis would also be sufficient to injure any or all of these structures.

Anatomic differences largely account for the disparity of incidences in urethral injuries in men and women. In men, the urethra is composed of anterior and posterior portions. The posterior portion is subdivided into membranous and prostatic urethra. The bladder neck and the prostatic and membranous urethra are relatively fixed in their positions to the pelvic ring by the puboprostatic ligaments. In females, the urethra is much shorter and more mobile, and urethral injuries are exceedingly uncommon.

Pelvic fracture occurs in 20 persons per 100,000 population. Motor vehicle accidents are by far the most common cause. Falls, athletic injuries, and industrial accidents are less common. Eighty five percent of noniatrogenic lower urinary tract traumatic injuries result from pelvic fractures. Conversely, approximately 25% of pelvic fractures have associated injuries to the urinary tract: 5–10% with urethral injuries and 5–15% with bladder injuries. Extraperitoneal bladder ruptures slightly exceed intraperitoneal ruptures. Combined urethral and bladder injuries occur approximately 1% of the time.

All patients with pelvis fractures should be considered to have associated bladder or urethral injury until proven otherwise. A thorough history of the incident, the sex of the patient, associated injuries, and hemodynamic stability of the patient should be taken into account. Urethral injury always should be suspected in men. Physical signs indicating urethral injury include blood at the meatus, gross hematuria, urinary retention, perineal or genital swelling, and abdominal tenderness. While the presence of any of these findings suggests injury, their absence does not rule it out. In fact, meatal blood—the most reliable indicator—may be absent up to 60% of the time. A high-riding prostate is nonspecific, difficult to demonstrate, and of limited diagnostic utility.

Since physical signs are not sensitive nor specific enough, radiographic assessments of all patients with pelvic ring fractures is indicated. In men, the retrograde urethrogram is the best and simplest test to rule out a urethral injury, and the threshold to perform this test should be low. Place an 18 or 20 Fr Foley catheter into the fossa navicularis, and inflate the balloon with 2–3 cc of saline to snug the catheter in place. Hold the penis on stretch at a perpendicular angle to the lower extremity. Inject 30–40 milliliters of contrast via a catheter tip syringe, and obtain an x-ray during the last 10 cc of injection. Extravasation without bladder filling indicates a complete disruption. Extravasation with bladder filling indicates partial disruption. If no injury or abnormality is demonstrated, the catheter may safely be passed into the bladder for both bladder drainage and evaluation of the bladder with a cystogram.

Cystograms should be performed on all patients with pelvic fracture. The critical aspects of cystograms are adequate filling and post-drainage images; 300 to 500 cc of contrast, infused under gravity, should be sufficient to demonstrate even small tears. A post-drainage film will demonstrate extravasation that had been masked behind the full bladder. Diagnostic findings of a teardrop bladder suggest pelvic hematoma.

Management of lower tract injuries may be divided into bladder and urethral injuries. In general, extraperitoneal bladder ruptures do not require surgical intervention. These patients may be cared for with catheter drainage for 7–10 days and antibiotics. A cystogram should be performed prior to removing the catheter to demonstrate adequate healing. Indications for surgery include exploration for associated injuries, removal of foreign bodies or bony spicules, and concomitant injuries to the bladder neck or urethra. Intraperitoneal bladder ruptures require operative repair. A lower midline vertical incision is used, which may be extended cephalad as other injuries dictate. Associated extraperitoneal injuries should be repaired from inside the bladder, and the bladder repaired with running 3-0 chromic suture in multiple layers. A large-caliber, 24–26 Fr Malecot suprapubic tube should be inserted through a different stab wound and left in place for 7–10 days in the absence of urethral injury.

Management of posterior urethral disruptions is more complicated and controversial. The debate pertains to immediate realignment versus open cystotomy tube with delayed urethroplasty. Immediate realignment sometimes avoids additional procedures, and if the procedures are still needed, they are technically less demanding. Critics argue that rates of restricture (up to 75%), impotence (30%), and incontinence (1.5%) are higher with immediate realignment. Immediate resuturing of the urethral ends is to be avoided as it is associated with 30% incontinence rates and 50–60% impotence rates. Current opinion in the debate suggests that it is the injury itself and not the repair method that results in impotence and incontinence. Delayed repair with open cystotomy allows for optimization of the patient's overall medical condition and more accurate radiographic assessment of length of the disrupted segment. Other minimally invasive techniques include "cut to the light" urethrotomies, core-through urethrotomies, and titanium stenting.

Initial management of pelvic fractures requires adherence to standard ATLS protocols. Assessment of airway, breathing, and circulation and an adequate primary survey will demonstrate any life-threatening injuries and should guide immediate treatment and resuscitation. The urologist enters the trauma evaluation during the secondary survey. Adequate treatment of lower urinary tract management is essential in minimizing long-term morbidity.

The present patient was brought into the trauma bay in severely critical condition. ATLS protocol was instituted immediately, with attention paid to immediate, life-threatening emergencies. In this man, hemorrhage was the most pressing problem and accounted for his hypotension, tachycardia, and probably mental derangement (although he also was intoxicated). Large-bore intravenous access was obtained, and massive volume resuscitation with crystalloid and blood started. According to ATLS guidelines, a Foley catheter may be passed via the urethra in the absence of urethral blood or a high-riding prostate; both were absent in this man. Thus, **a retrograde urethrogram** (RUG) was not performed. However, in pelvic fractures of this severity, with a wide diastasis of the pubic symphysis, a urethral disruption is likely. This patient did, in fact, have a urethral disruption, which was diagnosed intraoperatively when the catheter was seen in the pelvis, outside the urinary tract. For this reason, urologists recommend RUGs on all pelvic fracture cases prior to inserting the catheter.

Since pelvic fractures more commonly result in bladder injuries, ATLS protocol recommends cystograms for all pelvic fracture victims. Also, the absence of urine drained by the catheter in this patient prompted a cystogram to confirm placement of the catheter within the bladder. Another cause of his anuria may have been profound hypovolemia. Due to persistent hemodynamic instability and ongoing need for blood transfusion, he was taken to the operating room for pelvic fixation and exploratory laparotomy. In addition to his pelvic fracture and urethral injury, he had severe liver and splenic lacerations and a traumatic avulsion of his superior mesenteric artery. He died intraoperatively of massive, uncontrollable hemorrhage.

Clinical Pearls

1. All patients with pelvic fracture should be suspected of having a lower urinary tract injury.

2. Blood at the meatus may be absent in up to 60% of patients.

3. Extraperitoneal bladder rupture may be managed nonsurgically. Intraperitoneal rupture requires surgical repair.

4. In men, a Foley catheter should never be passed without a retrograde urethrogram.

5. If a cystotomy tube is needed in the trauma setting, it should be placed open under direct vision, not percutaneously.

REFERENCES
1. Spirnak JP: Pelvic fracture and injury to the lower urinary tract. Surg Clin North Am 68:1057–1069, 1988.
2. McAninch JW (ed): Traumatic and Reconstructive Urology. Philadelphia, W.B. Saunders Company, 1996.
3. Morey AF, McAninch JW: Reconstruction of posterior urethral disruption injuries: Outcome analyses in 82 patients. J Urol 157:506–510, 1997.
4. Zinman LM: Editorial: The management of traumatic posterior urethral distraction defects. J Urol 157:511–512, 1997.

PATIENT 52

A 54-year-old man with an elevated prostate specific antigen

A 54-year-old man is referred to your office with a PSA of 8 ng/ml, which was drawn by his internist on a routine annual visit. He has no urologic complaints. There is no history of urinary tract or prostate infection, erectile dysfunction, or recent urethral instrumentation. He has mild hypertension currently treated with both diet and exercise. The patient's father died at age 70 of prostate cancer.

Physical Examination: General: healthy appearing. Vital signs: normal. Chest: clear to auscultation and percussion. Cardiac: regular rate and rhythm, no evidence of murmur. Abdomen: soft, nontender, no evidence of distension, bowel sounds present. Genitourinary: normal circumcised phallus with palpably normal testes descended bilaterally. Digital rectal examination (DRE): 30-gram prostate (normal is approximately 20 grams) with normal anatomic landmarks, no evidence of palpable nodule or induration; normal anal sphincteric tone.

Laboratory Findings: WBC 4200/μl, hemoglobin 12.8 g/dl. BUN 15 mg/dl, creatinine 1.0 mg/dl. Urinalysis: specific gravity 1.010, pH 6.4, nitrite negative, leukocyte esterase negative, blood negative. Microscopic examination: 0–5 WBC/hpf, 0–5 RBC/hpf. Expressed prostatic secretion < 10 WBC/hpf. Urine culture: negative. Transrectal ultrasound–guided biopsy of the prostate: see figure.

Question: What is the etiology of this man's elevated PSA?

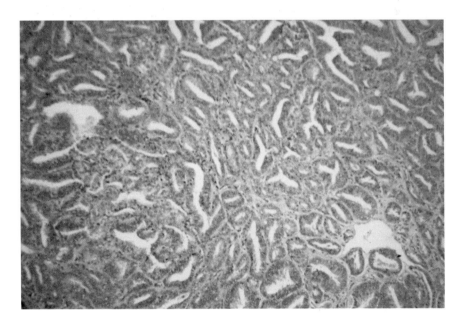

Diagnosis: Prostate cancer, stage T1c

Discussion: Prostate cancer remains the most common malignancy diagnosed in American men each year, with an estimated 300,000 new cases annually. Approximately 20% of all men diagnosed with prostate cancer succumb to the disease. The annual death rate of 38,000 men places this malignancy second only to lung in cancer-related deaths in American males. Men at a higher risk of having the disease include those with a family history and patients of African-American descent. Men with a first-degree relative diagnosed with prostate cancer run a greater than two-fold risk of being diagnosed with the disease. African-American patients have both a higher incidence and subsequent mortality, with an estimated 4.3% probability of dying from prostate cancer compared to 2.6% for white Americans.

Annual screening recommendations include serum PSA and DRE for all men over the age of fifty; screening should begin at age 40 for high-risk groups. Currently, the use of PSA in addition to DRE is the most cost-effective approach to screen men for prostate cancer. Although there are no data to suggest that overall survival of men with prostate cancer is improved with PSA screening, it is important to note that 60% of all newly diagnosed cancer is amenable to definitive localized therapy.

Since its widespread clinical acceptance approximately 10 years ago, PSA has become the most useful tumor marker in the field of oncology. PSA is an endogenous serine protease produced chiefly by the prostatic epithelium and to a lesser degree the periurethral glands. Its main known function is the liquefaction of the seminal coagulum in the ejaculate. Most of the circulating serum PSA is complexed largely to alpha 1 antichymotrypsin (an endogenous serine protease inhibitor) and, to a lesser degree, alpha 2 macroglobulin. Free or unbound PSA also exists, but in lower concentration than protein-bound PSA (usually < 30%). The half-life of serum PSA is approximately 2.5 days, and the normal range is 0–4 ng/ml.

The differential diagnosis of an isolated PSA elevation upon routine screening includes chronic bacterial prostatitis, iatrogenic or traumatic prostate manipulation, benign prostatic hyperplasia, and, most importantly, prostate cancer. The workup includes a thorough questioning to elicit any history of voiding symptoms, urinary tract infection, prostatitis, or recent urethral instrumentation. Physical examination should include a careful palpation of the prostate gland to determine size, symmetry, consistency, induration, and tenderness. The laboratory evaluation for an elevated PSA includes a complete urinalysis, voided urine culture, and examination of the expressed prostate secretion (EPS) for white blood cells. If the EPS contains > 10 WBC/hpf, then prostatitis is present and may be contributing to the elevated PSA. If the patient has or has had documented urinary tract infections, the prostate fluid should be cultured to rule out bacterial prostatitis (see table). If bacterial prostatitis is diagnosed, pathogen-specific treatment for 28 days with an oral fluoroquinolone or a 6-week regimen with trimethoprim/sulfamethoxazole is indicated. If the bacterial localization cultures do not yield an infectious etiology, the next step is transrectal ultrasound (TRUS)–guided needle biopsy of the prostate.

Four Glass Test for Urinary Bacterial Localization

Voided Urine Segment	Definition
VB1	Initial 10 cc voided urine
VB2	Midstream urine voided (clean catch sample)
EPS*	Prostatic secretions expressed during massage
VB3*	Voided urine after prostatic massage completed

VB = voided bladder urine, EPS = expressed prostatic secretions
* Physician-conducted prostatic massage

Sextant (six separate biopsy specimens) TRUS-guided biopsies using a spring-loaded, 18-gauge, hollow-bore needle secure adequate cores of prostate tissue for histologic diagnosis. Biopsies are taken from each lobe at the anatomic apex, at the mid portion of the prostate, and at the base of the peripheral prostatic zone. The peripheral zone of the prostate accounts for 75% of the gland's volume and is the location of approximately 70% of all adenocarcinoma of the prostate. In addition to sextant biopsies, all hypoechoic areas visualized on TRUS should be biopsied, as 33% of these areas harbor carcinoma. Major complications of office-based TRUS-guided biopsy include bleeding and urosepsis; however, both occur in less than 1% of patients if firm pressure is applied to the prostate after the biopsies and appropriate periprocedure antibiotics are used.

Approximately 95% of all prostatic adenocarcinomas are of an acinar cell origin. The Gleason grading system is used to assess tumor cell aggressiveness and clinical prognosis. Briefly, the grading system assigns a numerical value from 1–5 (grade 1 represents well-differentiated cells, whereas grade 5 is assigned to poorly differentiated tumor characteristics) for the predominant and the next most prevalent grade evident in the specimen. The final grade is the sum of the two numbers, and generally the higher this sum (grades 7–10), the worse the patient's chances for both organ-confined disease and overall disease-specific survival.

The TNM staging system for prostate cancer is shown at right. Treatment for stage T1c prostate cancer remains radical prostatectomy in a man with at least a predicted 10-year survival from other comorbidities. Alternative treatments include external beam radiotherapy, interstitial radioactive seed placement, cryoablation of the prostate, and watchful waiting. A pelvic lymph node dissection may be performed for clinical T1c prostate cancer, but the incidence of stage N1 disease (involved nodes) with a PSA < 10 ng/ml is less than 1%. Significant predictors of extracapsular or margin-positive disease (nonorgan-confined disease) for clinical T1c prostate cancer prior to radical prostatectomy are PSA and Gleason tumor grade by TRUS biopsy. The percentage of men with pathologically organ-confined prostate cancer after radical prostatectomy is 51–79% for clinical stage T1c disease; thus, an aggressive surgical approach is supported for this particular group of patients.

The present patient underwent TRUS-guided needle biopsy of the prostate, which revealed adenocarcinoma, Gleason grade 3 + 3. He underwent a radical retropubic prostatectomy without operative or postoperative complication. His final pathology was organ-confined disease to the prostate, Gleason grade 3 + 3.

TNM Clinical Staging System for Prostate Cancer

Clinical Stage	Description
T1a	Clinically unsuspected, incidental finding involving < 5% of specimen
T1b	Same as T1a but > 5% of specimen
T1c	Tumor identified on needle biopsy for elevated PSA
T2a	Palpable abnormality confined to prostate on DRE involving ≤ 50% of lobe
T2b	Same as T2a but involves > 50% of one lobe
T2c	Tumor palpated in both lobes
T3	Periprostatic disease extending through prostatic capsule into lateral sulcus of prostate or seminal vesicle
T4	Tumor fixed and invades adjacent structures other than seminal vesicle (e.g., bladder neck)
N1	Pelvic lymph node involvement
M1	Distant disease involving bone or other systemic areas

Clinical Pearls

1. Prostate cancer is the most common malignancy in American males, second only to lung in cancer-related mortality.

2. A combination prostate-specific antigen screening and digital rectal exam is the most cost-effective screening approach for prostate cancer.

3. PSA remains the most useful tumor marker in oncology.

4. TRUS-guided needle biopsy is used for definitive histologic diagnosis of prostate cancer. The peripheral zone of the prostate should be targeted on biopsy, as 70% of all adenocarcinoma originates in this area.

5. Approximately two-thirds of clinical T1c prostate cancer is pathologically organ-confined after radical prostatectomy, and this finding supports aggressive local management.

REFERENCES

1. Meares EM, Stamey TA: Bacteriologic localization patterns in bacterial prostatitis and urethritis. Invest Urol 5:492, 1968.
2. Silverberg E, Lubera JA: A review of American Cancer Society: Estimates of cancer cases and deaths. Cancer 36:9, 1986.
3. Hodge KK, McNeal JE, Terris MK, et al: Random systematic versus directed ultrasound-guided transrectal core biopsies of the prostate. J Urol 42:1008, 1989.
4. Walsh PC: Using prostate-specific antigen to diagnose prostate cancer: Sailing in uncharted waters. Ann Int Med 119:948, 1993.
5. Partin AW, Oesterling JE: Prostate-specific antigen in clinical urologic practice. AUA Update Series, Lesson 1, 1995.
6. Kozlowski JM, Grayhack JT: Carcinoma of the prostate. In Gillenwater JY, Grayhack JT, Howards SS, Duckett JW (eds): Adult and Pediatric Urology, 3rd ed. St. Louis, Mosby Year Book, 1996.
7. Cookson MS, Fair WR: Clinical stage T1c prostate cancer. AUA Update Series, Lesson 14, 1997.

PATIENT 53

A 27-year-old man with a scrotal mass

A 27-year-old white man presents with a 2-month history of a mass in the right hemiscrotum, which was discovered by his sexual partner. He describes the mass as firm and painless. He denies hematuria, dysuria, and urgency. He also denies any previous urinary tract infections or sexually transmitted diseases, and is otherwise in excellent health. He is not taking any medications.

Physical Examination: Temperature 36.6°; pulse 60; respirations 12; blood pressure 120/70. General: no apparent distress. Chest: clear. Abdomen: soft, nontender, no distension, normoactive bowel sounds. Genitourinary: penis circumcised; testes descended bilaterally with 2 × 2 cm, firm, painless mass in lower pole of right testis; mass does not transilluminate. Scrotum: normal. There is no evidence of inguinal or femoral hernia. Neurologic: normal.

Laboratory Findings: Electrolytes, BUN, creatinine: normal. CBC normal; serum lactate dehydrogenase 10/μl (normal 0–200); alpha-fetoprotein 0 ng/ml (normal 0–13); human chorionic gonadotropin 0 mIU/ml (normal 0–2). Chest radiograph: normal. Testicular ultrasound: see figure. Computed tomography scan of abdomen and pelvis: normal.

Question: What is the cause of the patient's scrotal mass?

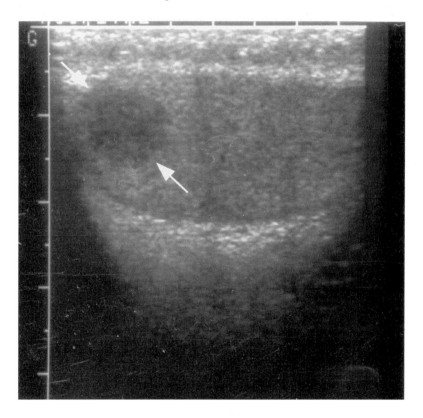

Diagnosis: Testicular seminoma

Discussion: Testicular cancer is a rare disease, with an incidence of only 2–3 new cases per 100,000 males reported in the United States each year. The lifetime probability of developing a malignant tumor of the testis is 0.2% for a white male in the U.S. Fortunately, as a result of advances in chemotherapy regimens, survival of patients with testicular cancer has dramatically improved.

The only known risk factors for testicular cancer are age, race, and cryptorchidism. Although testis cancer can occur at any age, the three peaks of incidence are 20–40 years of age, older than 60 years, and from birth until age 10. The incidence of testicular cancer in African-Americans is one-fourth that of whites. Finally, 10% of all testis tumors occur in undescended testes. The relative risk of malignancy is highest for the intra-abdominal testis (1 in 20) and significantly lower for the inguinal testis (1 in 80). However, 5–10% occur in the contralateral, normally descended testis.

Ninety-five percent of testicular tumors are germ cell tumors. Germ cell tumors of the testis tend to spread in a stepwise, lymphatic fashion. Because of their common embryologic origin with the kidney, testicular lymph nodes are concentrated at the level of the renal hilum, although they extend from T1 to L4. Accordingly, the primary landing site for the left testis is the left para-aortic area, and the primary landing site for the right testis is the right interaortocaval area.

Most testicular germ cell tumors present as a painless enlargement of the testis. Although most patients report a symptom duration of about 2.5 months, one-third present well after this time period, with a range up to 3 years. Indeed, testicular self-exam is an important screening tool to facilitate early diagnosis and successful treatment, as the length of delay correlates with the incidence of metastases. Approximately 10% of patients present with symptoms related to metastatic disease, including back pain, cough, dyspnea, bone pain, lower extremity swelling, anorexia, nausea, and vomiting.

Several tumor markers are important to the evaluation of a patient with testicular carcinoma, including alpha-fetoprotein (AFP), human chorionic gonadotropin (hCG), and lactate dehydrogenase (LDH). AFP is present in nonseminomatous germ cell tumors (NSGCT), but is never found in seminomas. Its half-life is 5 days. HCG, while more commonly elevated in NSGCTs, may be elevated in seminomas 7% of the time. HCG is classically elevated in choriocarcinoma. Its half-life is 1 day. LDH may be elevated in both NSGCTs and in seminomas.

Scrotal ultrasonography remains an important tool in differentiating between tumor and inflammatory disease. The technique also can be used to distinguish the tumor from epididymal pathology, and to evaluate the contralateral testis.

Exploration for a possible testis tumor includes inguinal exploration with cross-clamping of the spermatic cord vasculature. Radical orchidectomy is appropriate, as examination of the testis does not exclude cancer. Staging includes chest x-ray (posteroanterior and lateral) and CT of the abdomen and pelvis to assess the lungs and the retroperitoneum, the two most common sites of metastatic spread. The clinical stages for seminoma are: stage I—confined to the testis; stage II—regional lymph node spread (IIa is < 2 cm, IIb is > 2 cm); stage III—spread beyond regional nodes.

Low-stage seminoma (I, IIa) is extremely radiosensitive. Indeed, 95% of all stage I seminomas are cured with radical orchiectomy and retroperitoneal radiation. Further, low-volume retroperitoneal disease also is effectively treated with retroperitoneal irradiation, with an average 5-year survival rate of 87%.

Chemotherapy is used as salvage therapy for patients who relapse following irradiation. Patients with high-stage seminoma (IIb, III) or any seminoma associated with an elevated AFP should be treated with primary chemotherapy. Generally, seminomas are sensitive to platinum-based regimens, such as PVB (cisplatin, vincristine, and bleomycin). Ninety percent of patients with stage IIb or III disease have a complete response with chemotherapy.

In the present patient, an ultrasound showed a hypoechoic mass in the right testis. He underwent radical orchiectomy. Pathology confirmed the diagnosis of seminoma. Because of the negative chest x-ray and CT scan, the patient was determined to have stage I seminoma. He subsequently underwent retroperitoneal irradiation, and followup 1 year later showed no evidence of disease.

Clinical Pearls

1. The peak incidence of seminoma occurs between the ages of 20 and 40.

2. The most common histologically pure form of germ-cell tumor is seminoma, but mixed tumors occur more frequently than pure ones.

3. While cryptorchidism is an important risk factor for testis cancer, orchidopexy does not alter the malignant potential of the undescended testes; it merely facilitates examination and tumor detection.

4. The primary landing sites of testis cancer are the levels of the right interaortocaval area and the left para-aortic area.

5. Seminoma is exquisitely radiosensitive and chemosensitive.

REFERENCES

1. Donahue JP, Zachary SM, Maynard BR: Distribution of nodal metastases in nonseminomatous testis. J Urol 128:315, 1981.
2. Klein EA: Tumor markers in testis cancer. Urol Clin North Am 20:67–74, 1993.
3. Klein EA, Kay R: Testis cancer in adults and children. Urol Clin North Am 20(1), 1993.

PATIENT 54

A 34-year-old woman with the acute onset of hypertension

A 34-year-old white woman presents with the new onset of hypertension diagnosed on three separate blood pressure readings of 160/90 over the past month. The patient initially presented to her internist with a chief complaint of persistent headache. She denies any significant past medical or surgical history, and is currently on no medication. She smokes approximately one pack of cigarettes every week, and denies any family history of hypertension.

Physical Examination: General: appears comfortable. Temperature 37.1°; pulse 70; respirations 14; blood pressure 180/95 (lying), 175/90 (sitting). Chest: clear to auscultation and percussion. Cardiac: regular rate and rhythm, no evidence of murmur. Abdomen: soft, nontender, no masses palpated or percussed, bruit auscultated in left lower quadrant. Genitourinary: normal external genitalia; pelvic exam unremarkable.

Laboratory Findings: WBC 5400/μl, hemoglobin 12.9 g/dl, platelets 290,000/μl. Serum chemistry panel: Na^+ 137 mEq/L, K^+ 4.0 mEq/L, CO_2 24, BUN 12 mg/dl, creatinine 1.0 mg/dl. Urinalysis: specific gravity 1.010, pH 6.5, leukocyte esterase negative, nitrite negative, blood negative, human chorionic gonadotropin negative. Microscopic exam: no WBC or RBC. Plasma renin activity: baseline 4 ng/ml/hr; after single-dose (25 mg) captopril 18 ng/ml/hr. Differential renal vein renin sampling: right renal vein renin 6, left renal vein renin 15, vena cava renin 6. Selective renal artery arteriography: see figure.

Question: What is the etiology of this woman's hypertension?

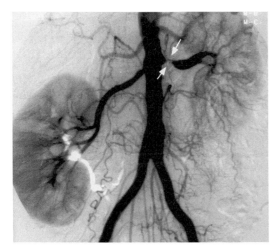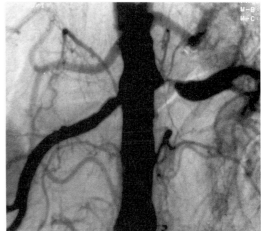

Diagnosis: Renovascular hypertension secondary to unilateral renal artery stenosis

Discussion: Hypertension affects approximately 60 million Americans, or 20% of the entire population. According to the ongoing research from the Framingham, Massachusetts study group, hypertension is the leading risk factor predisposing to heart attack, stroke, congestive heart failure, and renal failure. Hypertension is diagnosed as either primary or secondary. Essential or primary hypertension (hypertension of unknown etiology) accounts for 85–90% of all cases. Secondary (known) causes of hypertension that are part of the differential diagnosis include pheochromocytoma, adrenocortical disorders, thyroid disease, renal parenchymal disorders, obstructive uropathy, and renovascular hypertension. The latter accounts for roughly 5% of all cases. The definition of renovascular hypertension is a persistent hypertensive state (systolic pressure > 140 mmHg and diastolic > 90 mmHg) from a proven renal arterial lesion, usually > 70% obstruction.

Renovascular hypertension initially depends on increased renin secretion from the kidney that has the impaired blood flow, leading to angiotensin II formation and systemic arteriolar vasoconstriction. Thus, blood pressure becomes elevated secondary to the angiotensin II–induced vasoconstriction. Renin secretion from the opposite kidney remains suppressed. Ischemic nephropathy of the involved kidney results from the gradual loss of renal function, which is usually secondary to atherosclerotic renal vascular disease. Atherosclerosis accounts for approximately two-thirds of all cases of renovascular hypertension, and usually is diagnosed in elderly white males. Fibromuscular disease (mostly medial fibroplasia) accounts for the remaining cases, and is most commonly identified in white female patients in their third or fourth decade of life.

Risk factors that should alert the clinician to the possibility of renovascular hypertension include patients with a genetic predisposition, a history of cigarette smoking, and white race. Important clinical manifestations include an abrupt onset or exacerbation of hypertension with rapid progression, an abdominal bruit with both systolic and diastolic components, onset of hypertension before age 25 or after age 50, and inadequate blood pressure control with standard antiadrenergic agents or diuretic therapy. Because patients with renovascular hypertension have increased secretion of renin, **peripheral plasma renin activity** (PRA), when indexed versus the urinary sodium excretion rate, remains an excellent tool for identifying abnormally high renin secretion. Note that the blood used to determine peripheral PRA is collected at noon after 4 hours of patient ambulation.

The **single-dose captopril test** is a safe and inexpensive method for differentiating patients with renovascular hypertension from those with primary hypertension. The sensitivity and specificity of the single-dose captopril test is 100% and 95%, respectively—this is an excellent screening method for renovascular hypertension. The basis for this test is that angiotensin-converting enzyme (ACE) inhibitors produce a fall in blood pressure along with a marked rise in PRA in patients with renovascular hypertension. Patients must stop all antihypertensive medications, except beta blockers, 2 weeks before the test, and stay on a normal sodium diet. Criteria for a positive test that identifies a patient with renovascular hypertension are: (1) a post-captopril PRA > 12 ng/ml/hr, and (2) an absolute increase in renin of > 10 ng/ml/hr *plus* a 400% increase in renin if the baseline PRA was < 3 *or* a 150% increase in renin if the baseline was > 3 ng/ml/hr.

The effect of ACE inhibitors on patients with renovascular hypertension also is capitalized upon in the **captopril renogram**. This technique involves infusion of an ACE inhibitor to produce a dramatic fall in renal blood flow in the affected kidney by inhibiting the angiotensin II–induced efferent arteriolar constriction. The glomerular filtration rate in the kidney with the renal artery stenosis decreases, while the opposite kidney receives increased blood flow. The captopril renogram screening can be used to screen for renovascular hypertension, but it is more expensive than, and not as precise as, the single-dose captopril test. Duplex ultrasound of the renal arteries may be another noninvasive screening method; it is still under investigation.

Once a screening modality identifies renovascular hypertension, the physician may proceed to angiogram with or without differential renal vein renin determinations (RVR). An angiogram is performed immediately on patients at high risk, whereas patients with equivocal screening test results require RVR. Renal vein sampling after captopril stimulation increases renin release from the involved ischemic renal unit as compared to the contralateral renal unit and vena cava. Thus, localization of the involved renal unit is accomplished. If unequal, elevated renin levels, as compared to vena caval levels, are identified from both renal units, then the diagnosis of bilateral renal artery stenosis should be considered.

Renal arteriography is the gold standard for the definitive diagnosis and localization of renal artery stenosis. Some newer techniques being investigated and developed include spiral computed tomographic angiography and magnetic resonance angiography. This newer technology is advantageous because it is noninvasive.

Treatment options for patients with renovascular hypertension include medical antihypertensive therapy, surgical revascularization or nephrectomy, and percutaneous transluminal angioplasty (PTA). Patients treated medically, however, have a higher mortality, greater incidence of ischemic nephropathy, and less effective control of their blood pressure than those treated with surgical or PTA methods.

PTA is now the treatment of choice in most patients with fibromuscular hyperplasia, with success rates over 90%. Renal artery stents are used in conjunction with angioplasty when: (1) ostial lesions are present, (2) the lesion does not remain open after angioplasty, and (3) intimal tears occur during the procedure (stents can prevent secondary thrombosis).

In patients with atherosclerotic disease, PTA is not quite as successful (70–80% success rate), and surgical renal revascularization remains the primary intervention. The procedure of choice for open surgical revascularization is aortorenal bypass with autologous vein (usually saphenous). Current long-term success rates are as high as 90% in carefully selected patients with atherosclerotic disease.

In the present patient, RVR showed that left renal vein renin levels were supporting most of the peripheral renin. The renal angiogram demonstrated greater than 75% stenosis in the left renal artery. The patient underwent PTA and will return for followup shortly.

Clinical Pearls

1. Renovascular hypertension typically is characterized by stenosis of the renal artery from atherosclerosis or fibrous dysplasia.

2. Clinical tip-offs to the diagnosis include abrupt onset of hypertension and early or late age of onset.

3. The most useful screening tests for renovascular hypertension are measurement of peripheral plasma renin activity, the single-dose captopril test, and the captopril renogram.

4. Renal arteriography remains the gold standard for establishing the diagnosis of renal artery stenosis.

5. Treatment options for patients with renovascular hypertension include medical antihypertensive therapy, percutaneous transluminal angioplasty, and surgical revascularization or nephrectomy.

REFERENCES
1. Vaughan ED Jr, Buhler FR, Laragh JH, et al: Renovascular hypertension: Renin measurements to indicate hypersecretion and contralateral suppression, estimate renal plasma flow, and score for surgical curability. Am J Med 55:402, 1973.
2. Nally JV, Black HR: State-of-the-art review: Captopril renography—Pathophysiological considerations and clinical observations. Semin Nucl Med 22:85–97, 1992.
3. Schreiber MJ, Pohl MA, Novick AC: The natural history of atherosclerotic and fibrous renal artery disease. Urol Clin North Am 11:383–392, 1994.
4. Vaughan ED Jr, Sosa RE: Renovascular hypertension. In Walsh PC, et al (eds): Campbell's Urology, 7th ed. Philadelphia, WB Saunders Co, 1997.
5. Novick AC: Surgical correction of renovascular hypertension. Surg Clin North Am 68:1007, 1998.

PATIENT 55

A 58-year-old woman with low-grade fever, general malaise, and flank pain

A 58-year-old woman presented to her internist complaining of a 1-week history of worsening low-grade fevers, general malaise, and right flank pain. She had been "a bit under the weather" for several months, and her appetite had been poor during this time. The patient had lost 10 pounds in the last 3 months. Her urologic history includes recurrent episodes of cystitis, which have been treated empirically, as well as prior urologic instrumentation on one occasion. The patient also reports one episode of brief, total gross hematuria. She is otherwise healthy, and is taking only acetominophen at this time.

Physical Examination: Temperature 38.1°; pulse 100 and regular; other vital signs stable. Chest: clear. Abdomen: mildly distended, soft, with hypoactive bowel sounds. Spine: right costovertebral angle tenderness.

Laboratory Findings: WBC 12,400/μl, hemoglobin 9.8 g/dl (normocytic), BUN 15.2 mg/dl, creatinine 1.3 mg/dl. Sedimentation rate: elevated. Urinalysis: leukocyte esterase positive, nitrites positive, pH 8.0. Microscopic exam: hematuria, pyuria, and bacteriuria (see figure). Urine culture: pending.

Questions: What term describes the histologic process found within this patient's right kidney (shown in the figure)? What type of stones typically are associated with this disorder?

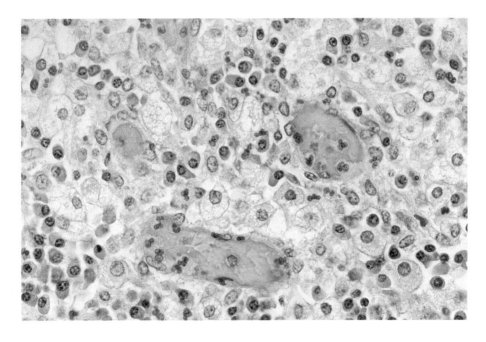

Diagnosis: Xanthogranulomatous pyelonephritis

Discussion: Xanthogranulomatous pyelonephritis (XGP), also known as replacement lipomatosis, was first described in 1916. It represents the end stage of a chronic renal inflammatory condition in which renal parenchyma undergoes lipomatous substitution with lipid-laden foamy macrophages (foam cells). If left unchecked, the process ultimately leads to extensive renal destruction and the production of a very large, nonfunctioning kidney. XGP generally is unilateral. There is an occasional association with renal cell carcinoma, and it often is difficult to exclude this possibility preoperatively based solely upon radiological and clinical grounds.

Lipomatous substitution of organ parenchyma with foam cells is not specific to the kidney. It is a process that occurs anywhere that chronic obstruction and infection/inflammation coexist. In the case of XGP, either a large renal pelvic or staghorn calculus almost uniformly causes the obstruction. The stones are typically triple-phosphate or calcium based. Other reported causes of renal obstruction include tumors, renal cysts, schistosomiasis, ureteropelvic junction obstruction, and reflux. Urine infection nearly always is present. The process of lipomatous substitution begins in the renal pelvis and progresses to include the calyces and parenchyma. Partial renal involvement has been reported in up to 20% of cases, especially in cases of renal duplication and in children.

Kidneys affected by XGP often are massively enlarged and distorted, yet the reniform outline is retained. Some degree of peri-pelvic fibrosis invariably is present, surrounding a stone-filled renal pelvis. This feature disallows the existence of massive pyelectasis. The calyces typically are filled with pus, and the cortex is filled with yellowish nodules that line the calyces. Histologically, these nodules are filled with foamy histiocytes intermixed with lymphocytes, multinucleated giant cells, and plasma cells. The lipid in foam cells consists of cholesterol esters and neutral fat that is thought to be the result of phagocytosis of lysed red blood cells.

The exact pathogenesis of XGP remains uncertain; however, it has been induced in an experimental rat model via the creation of infection and coincident chronic obstruction. Unproven hypotheses include abnormal lipid metabolism, lymphatic blockage, venous occlusion with resultant hemorrhage, and renal ischemia. Many of these patients have undergone prior urologic instrumentation (38%). In some way, XGP probably represents a morphologic and/or clinical variant of pyelonephritis.

XGP has been reported at nearly any age (1–87 years). The peak incidence occurs between the ages of 40 and 60; women are affected approximately three times more often than men. The typical presentation of XGP can include any combination of flank pain, fever, chills, malaise, weight loss, cystitis, anorexia, palpable mass, history of recurrent urinary tract infections, and hematuria. Renal cell carcinoma can present in much the same way, with the exception that the cancer patient typically exhibits fewer signs of an ongoing inflammatory condition.

Laboratory examination reveals anemia, leukocytosis, and elevated sedimentation rate. Fifteen percent of these patients are diabetic. Urinalysis reveals proteinuria and pyuria. The most common offending organisms found on urine culture are *Escherichia coli* (40%) and *Proteus* (30%); others include *Klebsiella* and *Pseudomonas*. One third of patients have sterile urine at the time of diagnosis due to pre-existing antimicrobial use. Azotemia or renal failure is uncommon because of the unilateral nature of this disorder. Interestingly, XGP is noted to cause reversible hepatic dysfunction in 20–40% of patients, leading to elevations in alkaline phosphatase, alpha-2-microglobulin, indirect bilirubin, and prothrombin time. These hepatic abnormalities reverse upon removal of the diseased kidney.

The best radiologic study for evaluating patients in whom XGP is suspected is computed tomography. The triad of enlargement, little to no function, and renal pelvic stone burden should be easily discernible. However, the identification of all three of these qualities simultaneously is quite variable. The calyceal nodules that are the pathologic hallmark of XGP do not enhance as tumors do. Radiologic evaluation typically generates a differential diagnosis including XGP (87% specific), renal cell carcinoma, malakoplakia in the absence of stone, and lymphoma. As renal cell carcinoma must be ruled out, the typical management plan involves partial or total nephrectomy. After nephrectomy, patients typically make a quick and full recovery. Recurrent XGP is exceedingly rare.

Although isolated, anecdotal success has been reported with approaches such as percutaneous nephrolithotomy and long-term intravenous antimicrobials, these should be considered only if nephrectomy would render the patient anephric. Otherwise, widespread experience suggests that antibiotics alone will not reverse the extensive loss of renal parenchyma typically seen in XGP. Likewise, mere incision and drainage is largely ineffective. Partial nephrectomy is being employed successfully in cases of segmental involvement. Ultimately, the diagnosis of XGP is a pathologic one.

The present patient was diagnosed by CT scan as having right renal duplication with lower-pole XGP, coincident with a lower-pole renal pelvic stone. A right lower-pole nephrectomy with reconstruction of the upper-pole ureter was performed. The patient quickly recovered and now is pain-free with sterile urine. She is being maintained on low-dose trimethoprim-sulfamethoxazole prophylactic therapy, twice daily.

Clinical Pearls

1. Patients with XGP typically present with indolent symptoms of chronic infection, including low-grade fever, malaise, and mild flank pain.

2. CT scan is the most useful and appropriate radiologic study to identify the typical triad of findings seen with XGP: renal enlargement, renal pelvic stone, and little to no function.

3. A minority of XGP patients (20–40%) exhibit hepatic dysfunction that reverses upon removal of the diseased kidney.

4. Treatment with antibiotics alone, resulting in eradication of infection, does not reverse the destruction of renal parenchyma caused by XGP.

5. Partial nephrectomy can be employed successfully in cases of segmental or focal XGP.

REFERENCES

1. Cohen MS:Granulomatous nephritis. Urol Clin N Amer 13(4):647–662, 1986.
2. Eastham J, Ahlering T, Skinner E: Xanthogranulomatous pyelonephritis: Clinical findings and surgical considerations. Urology 43(3):295–299, 1994.
3. Stam F, van den Tillaar PL, Falke TH, et al: Xanthogranulomatous pyelonephritis. Nephrol Dial Transplant 10(12):2365–2367, 1995.

PATIENT 56

A 26-year-old woman with urgency, frequency, and dysuria—third episode

A 26-year-old woman with no significant past medical history is referred for her third episode of urgency, frequency, dysuria, and sensation of incomplete emptying of the bladder (the latter symptom is of 1-year duration). At no time during these episodes has the patient experienced fever, chills, or flank pain. Each time, symptoms resolved after administration of a 3-day course of antimicrobials. The patient reports that her internist had diagnosed urinary tract infection via urine culture during one of the episodes. Even though she is asymptomatic for varying periods of time, the interval between symptomatic periods is becoming shorter. The patient is sexually active, and notes that her "infections" seem to correspond to periods of more frequent sexual activity. In fact, she states that she has had at least one of these infectious episodes every year since the onset of sexual activity. The patient's primary mode of contraception is a diaphragm used in conjunction with spermicidal jelly.

Physical Examination: General: well nourished, healthy appearing, no apparent distress. Vital signs: stable. Secondary sex characteristics: normal. Abdomen: soft; mild suprapubic tenderness upon palpation. Genitalia: normal; no adnexal fullness or tenderness, no discharge or cervical tenderness, urethra without mass or discharge upon "stripping."

Laboratory Findings: Urinalysis: positive for leukocyte esterase, nitrites, and leukocytes; 5–10 RBC/hpf, numerous WBC/hpf, heavy bacteriuria.

Questions: What further evaluation is needed? What is the appropriate categorization of this patient's urinary tract infections?

Diagnosis: Uncomplicated, recurrent cystitis

Discussion: Nearly half of all American women experience a urinary tract infection (UTI) at some point in their lifetime. Acute cystitis, defined as a nonspecific clinical syndrome usually consisting of dysuria, urinary frequency, urgency, and an occasional sensation of suprapubic fullness, is the most common form of UTI. This symptom complex is shared with other inflammatory conditions such as vaginitis, urethritis, interstitial cystitis, and urethral syndrome—as well as any condition characterized by urethral or pelvic discomfort. Therefore, it is important to distinguish the problem of acute cystitis from these other conditions early in the initial evaluation of a patient.

Evaluation of a patient with acute, recurrent cystitis should document infection, complicating factors that may warrant more intensive evaluation, and the pattern of infection recurrences. A simple or uncomplicated UTI is an infection in a normal urinary tract. A complicated UTI is an infection in a patient with structural or anatomic impairments that decrease the efficacy of antimicrobial therapy. Complicated infections often exhibit multidrug resistance, necessitate longer antimicrobial courses, and mandate more intensive urologic evaluation and treatment. Demonstration of poor empiric efficacy of initial antimicrobial therapy and development of fevers or generalized illness are indications of complication.

The patterns of infection may be subdivided into those that are isolated, unresolved, or recurrent. **Isolated infections** are the most common, occurring in 25–30% of women aged 30–40. They represent first infections or those that are spaced at least 6 months apart. **Unresolved infection** implies an attempt at treatment but an inability to effect sterile urine. Examples include pre-existing bacterial resistance, acquired resistance, urolithiasis, or inadequate antimicrobial coverage. **Recurrent infections** occur following documented successful resolution of an antecedent infection. If such an infection is new and has a point of origin outside the urinary tract, the term *reinfection* is applied (95% of all recurrent UTIs in women). If initial sterilization of the urine is followed by recurrence with the identical organism previously eradicated, the term *bacterial persistence* is applied. Persistent infections are often the result of anatomic abnormalities and are complicated. Radiologic and/or cytoscopic evaluation is warranted in these cases.

It is now clear that most women with reinfections have specific biologic phenotypes that promote ascending colonization and infection by promoting bacterial adherence to the vaginal, urethral, and bladder mucosa. Additionally, several behavioral risk factors for reinfections in women have been identified. Most clinicians empirically recognize that the onset of UTIs in women tends to coincide with the onset of sexual intercourse. Epidemiologic evidence of this includes the demonstration of increased bacteriuria after intercourse, the decreased risk of UTI in nuns, and the success of postcoital antimicrobial prophylaxis regimens. Use of the diaphragm also has been positively implicated. Contemporary studies specifically identify the use of spermicidal jelly with a diaphragm as being the most important factor, due to its promotion of vaginal colonization with *Escherichia coli.*

Evaluation should begin with a thorough history that is detailed enough to discern between acute cystitis and other causes of pelvic discomfort. A good history should elicit the presence of medical conditions that predispose to UTI (e.g., diabetes), as well as uncover the presence of childhood infections that suggest the presence of a congenital abnormality of the urinary tract. The possibility of complicating factors should lead to further radiologic or urologic evaluation. Also, the history can elicit the previous pattern of infections, the temporal relationship of infection to intercourse, and any culture records from prior episodes that would document infection and differentiate between reinfection and bacterial persistence.

After a vaginal examination to rule out gynecologic or urethral pathology, an in-office urinalysis is performed on a midstream voided or catheterized specimen. Results usually confirm the presence of cystitis (bacteriuria and pyuria), although low-count bacteriuria, for example at the onset of infection, may not be detectable microscopically. A simple, uncomplicated UTI can be treated empirically without a culture. In recurrent infections, it is important to establish the identity of the pathogen, so that when infections recur, differentiation can be made between persistence and reinfection. In a symptomatic patient, 10^2 cfu/ml is used as the cut-off for infection. Further radiologic or cystoscopic evaluation is reserved for patients in whom complicating factors, gross hematuria, fever, or flank pain is present, or for whom therapy is consistently ineffective.

Trimethoprim-sulfamethoxazole (TMP-SMX) is an excellent treatment choice for recurrent, simple infections. Fluoroquinolones should be reserved for complicated infections or resistant strains. A repeat urine culture should be obtained 7–10 days after treatment to document sterile urine or to define persistence.

In the present patient, there was no evidence that a complicating factor existed. Therefore, her infection was approached as an uncomplicated one. The pattern of infections was suggestive of recurrent infections, most likely due to reinfection, and a culture was performed for this reason. The culture revealed the presence of *E. coli*. Unfortunately, she likely will have recurrent infections throughout her life. The overall goal is to minimize the frequency of infections. Therefore, the patient was advised to discontinue use of the diaphragm/spermicidal jelly and switch to alternate forms of contraception. Given the close temporal relationship between intercourse and her cystitis, postcoital prophylaxis seemed to be the best initial strategy. After eradicating the *E. coli* UTI with a 3-day course of TMP-SMX, the patient began post-coital prophylaxis with a single dose of TMP-SMX. She since has suffered only one recurrent UTI after 2 years of followup. If reinfections continued to be a problem despite switching to different contraception, long-term TMP-SMX, nitrofurantoin, or cephalexin—daily or twice daily low-dose prophylaxis—would have been instituted.

Clinical Pearls

1. A thorough history and vaginal exam is essential when evaluating UTIs to differentiate cystitis from other causes of suprapubic discomfort in women.

2. Recurrent cystitis must be categorized as either reinfection or bacterial persistence before a proper long-term treatment plan can be formulated.

3. A 3-day course of antimicrobials is adequate to treat most uncomplicated cases of acute cystitis.

4. Recurrent UTIs should always be cultured before and after treatment for at least the first two to three episodes so that the infection pattern (reinfection versus persistence) can be established.

5. Radiologic or cystoscopic evaluation of recurrent UTIs should be reserved for patients in whom complicating factors, gross hematuria, fever, or flank pain is present, or for whom therapy is consistently ineffective.

6. Long-term strategies that have been effective in reducing the frequency of recurrent infection include chronic low-dose prophylaxis, self-start therapy, and postcoital prophylaxis.

REFERENCE
Hooton TM, Stamm WE: Management of acute uncomplicated urinary tract infection in adults. Med Clin North Am 75:339–348, 1991.

PATIENT 57

A 22-year-old woman with acute right flank pain and fever

A 22-year-old woman presents to the office with a 36-hour history of fever to 38.7°C and constant right-sided flank pain. She has had dysuria and foul-smelling urine for several days prior to the onset of pain. Although she admits to three episodes of cystitis per year for a period of 3 years, she has never had flank pain in the past. She does not complain of nausea, vomiting, or chills. She had been taking nitrofurantoin for this current episode, but without relief.

Physical Examination: General: appears uncomfortable. Temperature 38.2°; pulse 88; respirations 20; blood pressure 126/78. Back: right costovertebral angle tenderness. Remainder of physical exam: unremarkable.

Laboratory Findings: WBC 14,300/μl. Urinalysis: pH 6.9, 5–10 RBC/hpf, 50–100 WBC/hpf, many rods. Urine culture: pending.

Questions: Does this patient require hospitalization? What is appropriate followup?

Diagnosis: Acute uncomplicated pyelonephritis

Discussion: Acute pyelonephritis is an inflammation of the renal pelvis and kidney parenchyma that classically presents with fever, chills, and flank pain. Patients also may present with a number of less specific symptoms, such as nausea, vomiting, and diffuse abdominal pain, and a high index of suspicion must be maintained to make the diagnosis in these patients. As in infections of the lower urinary tract, acute pyelonephritis can be classified as complicated or uncomplicated based on the structural and functional integrity of the urinary tract.

Urinalysis in these patients usually demonstrates bacteriuria and pyuria. In 80% of community-acquired cases of pyelonephritis, *Escherichia coli* is the causative organism, with *Proteus, Pseudomonas, Enterobacter, Serratia,* and *Enterococcus* accounting for a majority of the remaining cases. Leukocytosis is common in the majority of immunocompetent patients. Blood cultures are not indicated unless the patient appears severely ill or is immunocompromised. Imaging studies, such as intravenous pyelogram, ultrasound, and CT scan, are used to rule out obstruction or identify a sequestrum of infection (i.e., abscess) that requires drainage. Imaging is required only for patients: who are initially septic-appearing, in whom obstruction is suspected, with a fever for longer than 3 days, and who do not respond to initial antimicrobial therapy.

A patient who presents with the classic symptoms of fever, chills, and flank pain and who is not septic or vomiting (as in this case) can be treated as an outpatient. Considering the typical causative organisms, trimethoprim-sulfamethoxazole (TMP-SMX) is the best first-line treatment. Fluoroquinolones also afford excellent coverage and tissue penetration, and they are an excellent option in the sulfa-allergic patient.

Patients who demonstrate clinical improvement within 72 hours of antimicrobial therapy should complete 14 days of therapy and then have repeat urine cultures to document cure. Lack of improvement within 72 hours or clinical deterioration at any time is an indication for hospitalization and intravenous treatment with broad-spectrum antimicrobials. If the patient does not improve with parenteral therapy or if symptoms persist for more than 7 days, perinephric abscess, obstruction, or unsuspected urinary tract abnormality should be considered.

This patient was started on oral TMP-SMX. Over the course of 24 hours, she became afebrile. After completing 14 days of therapy, she had a negative urine culture, which documented cure.

Clinical Pearls

1. A high index of suspicion is required to make the diagnosis, as not all patients present with the classic symptoms of fever, chills, and flank pain.
2. Imaging studies such as intravenous pyelogram, ultrasound, and CT scan are used if the clinical presentation suggests obstruction or fever has been present for longer than 3 days.
3. Patients that fit the clinical diagnosis and are not septic-appearing or vomiting may be treated on an outpatient basis.
4. Trimethoprim-sulfamethoxazole or a fluoroquinolone are excellent choices for empiric oral therapy of uncomplicated pyelonephritis.
5. Clinical deterioration or lack of improvement within 72 hours is indication for hospitalization, parenteral therapy, and imaging.

REFERENCE

Schaeffer AJ: Sections of the urinary tract. In Walsh P, Retik A, Vaughn ED Jr, Wein A (eds): Campbell's Urology, 7th ed. Vol. 1. Philadelphia, W.B. Saunders, 1997, pp 533–614.

PATIENT 58

A 74-year-old man with urinary intermittence and abdominal discomfort

A 74-year-old man presents with a chief complaint of urinary intermittence and lower abdominal discomfort that has been present for the last year. The patient has noted that his urinary stream abruptly stops and then resumes. His lower abdominal discomfort increases near the end of urination and is alleviated by lying flat on his back. He also has nocturia × 4 and has the sensation that he is not emptying his bladder even after double voiding. He was treated by his internist for a culture-documented *Escherichia coli* urinary tract infection 2 months ago. (No post-antimicrobial cultures were sent.) There is no history of prior urologic surgery and, other than mild hypertension that is controlled by a calcium channel blocker, he has no medical illnesses.

Physical Examination: Temperature 37.2°. Abdomen: bladder vaguely palpable (gives patient sense of needing to void). Rectal exam: prostate approximately 60 g; prostate surface without induration, landmarks intact.

Laboratory Findings: Urinalysis: 50–100 RBC/hpf, numerous WBC/hpf, bacteria. Urine culture: *E. coli* 10^5 cfu/ml. Abdominal ultrasound: no hydronephrosis; approximately 300 cc post-void residual; three mobile filling defects with dense shadowing.

Question: What is your diagnosis?

Diagnosis: Bladder stones secondary to chronic urinary obstruction

Discussion: The composition, etiology, and age distribution of patients with bladder calculi varies around the world. In the United States, uric acid stones represent over 50% of bladder calculi, with struvite also making up a large percentage. Calcium oxalate bladder stones often herald an upper tract origin. The predominant cause of bladder calculi is bladder outlet obstruction, usually from benign prostatic hyperplasia. In North America, primarily adults are afflicted with bladder stones; in other parts of the world, where malnutrition is more rampant, children also are affected. When patients with obstructive symptoms were studied with intravenous pyelogram or ultrasound in large series, 2.7–3.2% were found to have bladder stones. In the asymptomatic population, the proportion with bladder stones was only 0.1%. Routine radiographic evaluation for bladder stones is not recommended unless there is strong clinical suspicion.

Treatment of bladder calculi has two main goals: first, to completely remove all stone material; second, to correct the defect that caused the stones to form. In addition to open cystolithotomy, there are numerous endoscopic methods available for stone removal. Consider the stone burden before recommending a procedure. If the stone burden is large, then cystolithotomy is preferable to a prolonged endoscopic procedure. For small stones, endoscopic methods such as electrohydrolic lithotripsy, ultrasound, or a variety of lasers are effective. Endoscopic techniques can be performed under local anesthetic or intravenous sedation. Once the patient has been rendered stone-free, the underlying cause of stone formation should be identified and corrected. In many instances the cause is bladder outlet obstruction secondary to benign prostatic hyperplasia.

In the present patient, bladder outlet obstruction and the presence of benign prostatic hyperplasia had resulted in the formation of three small stones, which were revealed on the ultrasound. The urinary tract infection was treated with a fluoroquinolone, and the patient was maintained on therapy to ensure no growth during surgery. He underwent an electrohydrolic lithotripsy and a transurethral resection of his prostate. The resection was performed to relieve the obstruction and reduce the likelihood of stone recurrence. Typically, bladder stones forming as the result of bladder outlet obstruction are composed of uric acid.

Clinical Pearls

1. The diagnosis of bladder stones often depends on a high index of suspicion and a thorough history.

2. Benign prostatic hyperplasia is the most common cause of bladder stones in North America.

3. Uric acid and struvite stones comprise the majority of bladder stones.

4. Electrohydrolic lithotripsy, ultrasound, a variety of lasers, and open surgery are all options for the treatment of bladder stones.

5. Correcting the underlying pathology (e.g., transurethral prostatectomy for benign prostatic hyperplasia) is essential for complete treatment of patients with bladder stones.

REFERENCES

1. U.S. Department of Health and Human Services: Benign Prostate Hyperplasia: Diagnosis and Treatment. AHCPR Pub. No. 94-0582. Clinical Practice Guideline. Washington DC, DHHS, 1994.
2. Menon M, Parulkar BG, Drach GW: Urinary lithiasis: Etiologies, diagnosis, and medical management. In Walsh P, Retik A, Vaughan ED Jr, Wein A (eds): Campbell's Urology, 7th ed. Vol. 3. Philadelphia, W.B. Saunders, 1997, pp 2661–2733.

PATIENT 59

A 21-year-old woman with urgency, frequency, and dysuria—
first episode

A 21-year-old woman seeks urologic evaluation for a 3-day history of dysuria. She also is urinating frequently (every 1–2 hours) and experiencing a sense of urgency and incomplete emptying. She denies a previous similar episode at any point in her life and also denies any prior surgeries, fevers, flank pain, and hematuria. She takes no medications and is sexually active with a single partner.

Physical Examination: General: appears well. Temperature 36.8°; pulse 72; respirations 14; blood pressure 112/64. Abdomen: some mild suprapubic tenderness. Back: no costovertebral angle tenderness. Genitalia: no lesions, no cervical motion tenderness, no adnexal masses or tenderness.

Laboratory Findings: Urinalysis: 0–5 RBC/hpf, numerous WBC/hpf, bacteria.

Questions: What are important points to establish by history? What constitutes appropriate therapy?

Diagnosis: Acute uncomplicated bacterial cystitis

Discussion: Cystitis, an infection of the urinary bladder, affects 4–6 million women and prompts approximately 7 million office visits each year. In the 20- to 40-year-old age group, approximately 25% of women will experience at least one urinary tract infection (UTI).

A thorough history is imperative in generating an appropriate differential diagnosis and in directing therapy. Conditions such as bacterial vaginosis, sexually transmitted diseases, interstitial cystitis, and other noninflammatory conditions, all of which have different treatments, usually can be separated based on the history. It is also important to elicit any history of previous UTI, as well as any factors that can initiate (e.g., urethral catheterization or sexual intercourse) or complicate (e.g., diabetes mellitus or pregnancy) a UTI.

Classification of the type of infection is important and typically is divided between uncomplicated and complicated. An **uncomplicated** urinary tract infection is one that occurs in a patient whose urinary tract is normal from both a structural and functional perspective. It follows that a patient with a **complicated infection** has either structural or functional abnormality of their urinary tract. Further divisions include isolated infection, unresolved infection, and recurrent infection, which is subsequently divided into reinfection or bacterial persistence. *Isolated* infections are either initial infections or those separated from another episode by 6 months. Isolated infections account for 25–40% of infections in women. *Unresolved* infections occur in patients in whom antimicrobial therapy has been unsuccessful. *Recurrent* infections are either reinfections representing discrete episodes of infection that are initiated from outside the urinary tract, or bacterial persistence, which is indicative of a site of bacterial sequestration that has been protected from antimicrobial therapy. Recognizing bacterial persistence is important as the cause must be removed to allow successful therapy.

If the patient has a history that is consistent with an uncomplicated UTI, it is not necessary to obtain a urine culture as long as the patient responds to appropriate empiric therapy. If the patient does not respond to therapy, then a urine culture should be obtained, and the therapy should be broadened until it can be tailored based on the culture and sensitivity results. Routine pretreatment cultures have been shown to increase cost by 40% while only decreasing overall symptom duration by 10%. As 85% of community-acquired urinary tract infections are caused by *Escherichia coli*, trimethoprim-sulfamethoxazole (TMP-SMX) is an excellent choice for empiric therapy. For an uncomplicated UTI in a female patient, 3 days of therapy is sufficient, and a followup urinalysis should be obtained 7–10 days after therapy to document cure. Fluoroquinolones should be reserved for those with complicated or recurrent infections, allergy to TMP-SMX, or resistant organism.

If the patient has a poor response to therapy or subsequent infections, further urologic evaluation may be warranted. If her history reveals a relationship between reinfections and sexual intercourse or her menopausal status, then pericoital prophylaxis or estrogen replacement therapy should be considered.

The present patient was treated with a 3-day course of TMP-SMX and responded to therapy. She noted no relation to intercourse and never had a repeat episode. The diagnosis was arrived at by exclusion. If recurrence is a problem, or the patient develops fever or sepsis, a more intensive evaluation is required.

Clinical Pearls

1. A thorough history coupled with a urinalysis that reveals pyuria and bacteriuria can allow a presumptive diagnosis of UTI.

2. Urine culture, which is the gold standard for assessing infection, is not always required for isolated, presumably uncomplicated UTIs in women.

3. The standard threshold to diagnose infection is lowered to 10^2 cfu/ml in symptomatic patients.

4. A 3-day course of TMP-SMX is adequate therapy for most uncomplicated UTIs.

5. Followup urinalysis should be obtained 7–10 days post therapy to document cure.

6. Recurrent infections that have a relationship to sexual intercourse or estrogen depletion may be reduced by pericoital antimicrobial prophylaxis or estrogen replacement therapy, respectively.

REFERENCE

Schaeffer AJ: Sections of the urinary tract. In Walsh P, Retik A, Vaughan ED Jr, Wein A (eds): Campbell's Urology, 7th ed. Vol. 1. Philadelphia, W.B. Saunders, 1997, pp 533–614.

PATIENT 60

A 48-year-old woman with urinary incontinence

A 48-year-old woman is seeking evaluation for urinary incontinence. She underwent surgical treatment for stress urinary incontinence 5 years ago, which initially was successful. However, over the last year she has developed recurrent incontinence. Leakage is associated with coughing, sneezing, and heavy lifting, and she now requires one or two pads per day to prevent soiling her clothes. Other voiding symptoms consist of occasional urgency and daytime frequency (every 2 hours). She reports no urge incontinence, nocturia, hematuria, dysuria, hesitancy, post-void dribbling, or sense of incomplete emptying.

The patient has borne four healthy children. Her last menstrual period was 2 weeks ago. She denies a history of urinary tract infections, neurologic disease, additional pelvic surgery, or diabetes. She takes no medications. She is a homemaker and works part-time as a nurse. A 24-hour voiding diary obtained prior to the clinic visit demonstrated a functional bladder capacity of 350 cc, normal 24-hour urine output, and three episodes of medium-volume stress incontinence.

Physical Examination: Vital signs: normal. Abdomen: soft; no masses or tenderness; no peripheral edema. Genitalia: normal; no cervical motion tenderness or adnexal masses; mild (Grade I) cystocele, no enterocele or rectocele; normal pelvic muscle contraction. Rectum: normal anal sphincter tone, perineal sensation, and bulbocavernosus reflex. Catheterized post-void residual: 20 cc. Swab test: 45° rotation. After filling the bladder to 200 cc, coughing produces a 2-inch stream of leakage from the urethra.

Laboratory Findings: CBC, serum electrolytes, BUN, creatinine, fasting blood sugar: normal. Urinalysis: 0–2 WBC/hpf, 0 RBC/hpf, no bacteria, rare epithelial cells. Urine culture: negative.

Question: Describe the basic workup for female urinary incontinence.

Answer: The basic workup includes a thorough history (including 24-hour voiding diary with or without pad test), urinalysis, and physical examination (may include swab test or cystometrogram).

Discussion: An estimated 10 million Americans suffer from urinary incontinence, including up to 50% of elderly, institutionalized individuals. Among the female population between 30 and 59 years of age, approximately 15% perceive incontinence as a social problem. The total annual cost to society is estimated at 10 billion dollars. All physicians who care for adult patients should be prepared to evaluate and treat the common causes of urinary incontinence.

Normal bladder function consists of a filling phase and an emptying phase. Filling is characterized by a low intravesical pressure, a closed bladder neck, and absence of involuntary bladder contractions. Voiding consists of a coordinated, sustained detrusor contraction with simultaneous relaxation of the bladder neck and urethral sphincter. Anatomic obstruction must be absent for effective voiding to occur. Each type of voiding dysfunction can be categorized as either a failure to empty or a failure to store, and subcategorized as due to dysfunction of either the bladder or urethra. Incontinence represents a failure to store urine adequately. Urge incontinence is a failure to store due to the bladder, and stress incontinence is a failure to store due to the outlet. Sometimes the two coexist in a given patient.

Urge incontinence refers to leakage caused by involuntary bladder contractions. In the presence of neurologic disease, such involuntary contractions are referred to as *detrusor hyper-reflexia*; in the absence of overt neurologic pathology, they are called *detrusor instability*. Common causes of urge incontinence include upper motor neuron lesions, such as in stroke and Parkinson's disease, and inflammatory lesions in the bladder, such as those resulting from cystitis, carcinoma in situ, and bladder stones. In the elderly, uninhibited detrusor activity can result from transient causes.

Stress incontinence results from defective urethral sphincter function. Leakage may result from a weakening of the pelvic support structures due to aging or multiparity. When this weakening occurs, the proximal urethra and bladder neck descend abnormally during straining, and urine is forced out. Such stress incontinence due to *urethral hypermobility* is usually mild. More severe degrees of stress incontinence generally result from damage to the urethral sphincter. This type of stress incontinence is referred to as *intrinsic sphincter deficiency*, and is frequently associated with prior pelvic surgery, trauma, or radiation.

The purpose of the evaluation of the incontinent female patient is to locate the abnormality (bladder, urethra, or both) and determine its severity. From this information, the exact etiology is inferred, and a rational treatment plan can be initiated. The evaluation begins with a careful history. Daytime and night-time frequency of urination should be determined. The exact nature of the patient's symptoms should be ascertained, including the frequency, volume, timing, and duration of incontinence. Presence of irritative symptoms (e.g., frequency, urgency, nocturia, dysuria) and obstructive symptoms (e.g., hesitancy, decreased force of stream, sense of incomplete emptying, post-void dribbling) are also significant.

A more objective evaluation of the incontinence may be obtained via a 24-hour voiding diary. The patient is asked to record the time of day and volume of each void, as well as the timing and estimated volume (small, medium, large) of each incontinence episode. Total fluid intake also may be recorded. Information obtained with the voiding diary includes total voided volume, functional bladder capacity (largest voided volume during the 24-hour period), frequency of micturition, diurnal urine output, frequency of leakage, and association of leakage with stress or urge episodes. The voiding diary is an invaluable tool in assessing patterns of incontinence. For some patients, simply voiding more frequently to keep bladder volumes below their "leak threshold" will result in dryness.

Another more objective evaluation of the degree of incontinence is the 24-hour pad test. This involves the collection of all incontinence pads used by the patient for a 24-hour period. The pads are weighed to assess the degree of leakage (1 gram = 1 cubic centimeter). Alternatively, the patient may be prescribed phenazopyridine, which turns the urine orange-colored. The amount of staining on the pads can be used to estimate the severity of the incontinence.

A focused past medical history should be obtained in all patients. Neurologic diseases such as multiple sclerosis, spinal cord injury, back surgery, Parkinson's disease, stroke, and myelodysplasia may affect bladder or sphincter function. Prior pelvic surgery may injure pelvic nerves controlling micturition. Numerous vaginal deliveries cause local tissue damage which may contribute to the incontinence. The date of the last menstrual period should be obtained, as lack of estrogen in postmenopausal women causes urethral mucosal atrophy and consequent poor tissue apposition.

Reviewing patients' medications and allergies may provide insight into prior or current therapy for the incontinence. Anticholinergic medications used to treat urge incontinence often are poorly tolerated due to side effects, causing patients to list them as allergies. Some other medications even can contribute to incontinence, especially in elderly patients.

Prior to physical examination, a voided specimen is obtained for urinalysis. If the voided specimen contains numerous vaginal epithelial cells, a catheterized specimen is obtained during the physical examination.

The physical examination begins with an assessment of gait and mobility. The abdomen is examined for masses, tenderness, and bladder distention. Lower extremity strength, sensation, and reflexes are assessed. Signs of fluid overload such as peripheral edema are noted. A regional neurologic evaluation of the sacral dermatomes is performed by evaluating anal sphincter tone, perianal sensation, and presence of the bulbocavernosus reflex. The latter is checked by quickly squeezing the clitoris or lightly tugging on an indwelling Foley catheter and feeling a contraction of the anal sphincter around the examiner's finger.

Pelvic examination is performed to check for masses or pelvic prolapse (e.g., cystocele, rectocele, enterocele, or uterine prolapse). Urethral mobility may be evaluated with the **swab test**. A lubricated, sterile swab is inserted into the urethra. The patient is asked to strain, and the degree of rotation is observed. A rotation of greater than 30 degrees is indicative of urethral hypermobility. Urethral catheterization is performed, and the postvoid residual is determined. The bladder then is filled to 200 cc. Repeat pelvic examination with the bladder filled may demonstrate a cystocele that was not previously evident. The patient is asked to cough or strain and the presence and degree of stress-induced leakage is noted. If no leakage occurs despite a clear history of stress incontinence, the exercise may be repeated with the patient standing.

In patients with symptoms of urge incontinence, a bedside **cystometrogram** may be performed. After urethral catheterization, a 60-cc catheter-tipped syringe is attached to the Foley catheter and the plunger of the syringe is removed. Sterile saline or water is poured into the open syringe, which is held approximately 20 centimeters above the bladder. The bladder slowly is filled, and the patient reports the first sensation of bladder filling, first desire to void, and first sense of urgency. The volumes at which these sensations occur are noted. Delayed sensation of filling may indicate underlying neurologic pathology. A sudden rise in the level of the fluid meniscus in the absence of an increase in abdominal pressure generally indicates an uninhibited detrusor contraction.

In the elderly, particular attention should be directed to identifying potential causes of **transient incontinence**. Transient incontinence refers to leakage caused by potentially reversible conditions rather than underlying pathology. It generally manifests as urge incontinence or overflow incontinence (leakage due to a chronically overfilled bladder). The eight causes of transient incontinence can be remembered with the mnemonic DIAPPERS: Delirium, urinary tract Infection, Atrophic vaginitis, Pharmaceuticals (particularly narcotics, anticholinergics, sedatives, and psychotropic medications), Psychogenic causes, Excess urine output due to polydipsia or diuretic use, Restricted mobility, and Stool impaction.

Further evaluation with imaging studies and/or cystoscopy is reserved for patients with hematuria, persistent infections, or suspected tumor or bladder stone.

After the basic evaluation outlined above has been completed, the type of incontinence often is well defined. At other times, the initial evaluation is inconclusive, and more sophisticated **urodynamic studies** are necessary. Formal urodynamic evaluation also is indicated when initial treatment has been unsuccessful; following failed corrective surgery; in patients with neurologic disease; and in patients with a history of radical pelvic surgery. These studies rely on a urodynamics laboratory equipped to measure simultaneous abdominal and bladder pressures during filling and voiding, sphincter EMG activity, urinary flow rate, and urethral pressure. Instead of water or saline, the bladder may be filled with contrast material; fluoroscopic evaluation of the lower urinary tract is then possible. Urodynamic data may be helpful in determining the etiology of a patient's stress incontinence by determining the bladder pressure at which leakage occurs (leak point pressure). If leakage occurs at a pressure of greater than 90 cm H_2O, urethral hypermobility is the cause. If leakage occurs at a pressure below 60 cm H_2O, intrinsic sphincter deficiency exists. Leakage between these two values indicates a combination of the two mechanisms.

Treatment of incontinence can be divided into three categories: rehabilitative, pharmacologic, and surgical. Unless the problem is quite severe, initial treatment is nonsurgical. For urge incontinence, rehabilitative techniques consist of timed voiding, adjustment of fluid intake and diuretic use, and Kegel exercises to improve pelvic floor strength and thus suppress involuntary bladder contractions. Transient factors that may be contributing to the incontinence also must be addressed. Pharmacologic treatment with anticholinergic agents (e.g., oxybutinin, propantheline) or tricyclic antidepressants (e.g., imipramine) is common. These agents cause an increase in the volume at which an uninhibited contraction occurs, but generally do not abolish such contractions. Thus, it is essential to continue timed voiding in patients treated with these drugs. Anticholinergic side effects are common, especially in the elderly. Surgical treatment generally is reserved for patients with overt neurologic disease, severe detrusor hyper-reflexia, and low-capacity, low-compliance bladders. Such treatment consists of augmentation cystoplasty or urinary diversion.

For stress urinary incontinence, rehabilitative techniques are similar to those used for urge incontinence. However, the emphasis in these patients is to teach selective contraction of the pelvic floor muscles (**Kegel exercises**) without simultaneously increasing intra-abdominal pressure. Patients may learn to isolate these muscles by voluntarily interrupting the urinary stream. In patients who have difficulty with this, further instruction with biofeedback training or electrical stimulation may be necessary. Pharmacologic agents play less of a role in the treatment of stress incontinence than urge incontinence. In peri- or postmenopausal women with mild stress incontinence, estrogen administration may diminish incontinence by improving urethral closure. Nonsurgical management of stress incontinence is rarely curative except in the most mild of cases.

Some women are content with the improvement obtained by such conservative measures. The remainder require surgery. For urethral hypermobility, surgery consists of suspending the periurethral tissues from the rectus fascia so that a "hammock" of supporting tissue is created beneath the urethra (bladder neck suspension). This can be accomplished via a transvaginal approach (Raz, Stamey, Pereyra procedures) or an open, retropubic approach (Marshall-Marchetti-Krantz, Burch procedures). For intrinsic sphincter deficiency, urethral coaptation must be surgically enhanced. This can be done with submucosal collagen injections performed through the cystoscope, or with placement of a fascial strip immediately beneath the urethra, which is suspended from the rectus fascia (pubovaginal sling). Recent data has called into question the long-term durability of the bladder neck suspension procedures. Therefore, some surgeons treat all types of female stress incontinence with a sling procedure.

The present patient was not interested in conservative treatment for her incontinence because she wished to resume an active lifestyle. The swab test was consistent with recurrent urethral hypermobility. Urodynamic evaluation demonstrated a leak point pressure of 80 cm H_2O, indicating a component of intrinsic sphincter deficiency. She underwent pubovaginal sling placement, and had no further problems with incontinence.

Clinical Pearls

1. Detrusor instability refers to uninhibited detrusor contractions in a neurologically intact patient; detrusor hyper-reflexia refers to such contractions in a patient with neurologic disease.

2. The causes of transient incontinence include Delirium, urinary tract Infection, Atrophic vaginitis, Pharmaceuticals, Psychogenic causes, Excess urine output, Restricted mobility, and Stool impaction (DIAPPERS).

3. A voiding diary is an essential part of the workup of an incontinent female patient.

4. Incontinence associated with prior pelvic surgery, trauma, or radiation may be due to intrinsic sphincter deficiency.

5. Formal urodynamic evaluation is indicated when the etiology of the incontinence is unclear; after initial treatment has been unsuccessful; following failed corrective surgery; in patients with neurologic disease; and in patients with a history of radical pelvic surgery.

REFERENCES
1. Resnick NM: Voiding dysfunction in the elderly. In Yalla SV, McGuire EJ, Elbadawi A, Blaivas JG (eds): Neurourology and Urodynamics. New York, MacMillan Publishing Co., 1988, pp 303–330.
2. Bushman W: Evaluation and treatment of urinary incontinence in the adult. Compr Ther 20:224–231, 1994.
3. Klutke CG, Raz S (eds): Evaluation and treatment of the incontinent female patient. Urol Clin North Am 22:481–697, 1995.
4. Blaivas JG, Romanzi LJ, Heritz DM: Urinary incontinence: Pathophysiology, evaluation, treatment overview, and nonsurgical treatment. In Walsh PC, Retik AB, Vaughan ED, Wein AJ (eds): Campbell's Urology, 7th ed. Philadelphia, W.B. Saunders, 1998, pp 1007–1043.

PATIENT 61

A 72-year-old woman with microscopic hematuria

A 72-year-old woman with hypertension and diabetes is referred by her internist for persistent microscopic hematuria. A routine urinalysis obtained by the internist 2 weeks ago demonstrated 5–10 RBC/hpf. Urine culture was negative. She denies a history of irritative or obstructive voiding symptoms, flank pain, nephrolithiasis, and urinary tract infections. Past surgical history is remarkable for a cholecystectomy and total abdominal hysterectomy for uterine leiomyomas. Her medications are Lasix, Premarin, and Glyburide. She has a 35 pack-year smoking history, and she is a retired homemaker. There is no family history of nephrolithiasis.

Physical Examination: Temperature 37.1°, pulse 80, respirations 18, blood pressure 140/88. General: mildly obese; appears comfortable. Abdomen: soft, no masses or organomegaly; surgical incisions well-healed. No flank or suprapubic tenderness. Genitalia: normal. Bimanual exam: no masses; cervix surgically absent.

Laboratory Findings: Current office urinalysis: 5–10 RBC/hpf, 0–2 WBC/hpf, no bacteria, no epithelial cells. Urine culture: negative. CBC: normal. BUN and creatinine: normal. Urine cytology: negative. Cystoscopy: 1-cm papillary lesion just lateral to left ureteral orifice (see figure).

Question: What is your diagnosis?

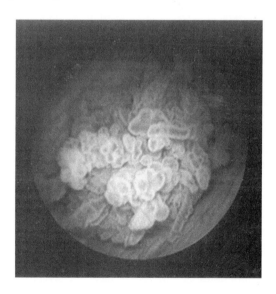

Diagnosis: Transitional cell carcinoma, superficial

Discussion: Hematuria is one of the most common causes for urologic referral. Greater than 3 RBC/hpf on a properly obtained urinalysis is considered significant and mandates evaluation of the urinary tract. The risk of a life-threatening condition increases with the degree of hematuria. However, tumors may be found in as many as 10% of patients presenting with asymptomatic microscopic hematuria.

The most common urologic causes of hematuria include tumors, urolithiasis, urinary tract infections, and benign prostatic hyperplasia. In younger patients, infections and stones frequently are found, while bladder tumors are the most frequent source of gross hematuria in patients over the age of 50. Other causes of hematuria include medical renal diseases, trauma, sickle-cell disease, exercise-induced hematuria, hypercalciuria, and renal vein thrombosis. A thorough history, physical examination, and urinalysis will provide significant clues as to the source of the blood, but definitive evaluation requires upper tract imaging and lower tract endoscopy. Hematuria in the adult should be considered indicative of malignancy until proven otherwise. Accordingly, the workup should be carried out in an expedient manner.

The history should include a determination of the degree and timing of the hematuria. Gross hematuria is evident to the naked eye; microscopic hematuria is seen only under the microscope. It is common for an initial episode of gross hematuria to be followed by persistent microscopic hematuria. Gross hematuria can be further classified according to its timing during the urinary stream. Initial hematuria indicates a urethral source; terminal hematuria indicates disease in the bladder neck or prostatic urethra; total hematuria indicates a bladder or upper tract source. Presence of large clots indicates significant bleeding, which may cause urinary retention, while vermiform clots typically originate in the ureters or kidneys.

All patients should be asked about the presence of pain or coexisting voiding symptoms. Dull flank pain may be caused by a renal mass. Colicky flank pain frequently indicates the presence of an obstructing ureteral stone or blood clot. Suprapubic discomfort, frequency, and urgency may indicate a urinary tract infection or presence of carcinoma in-situ (CIS) in the bladder.

A thorough past medical history can give important clues as to the source of the hematuria. Recent urinary tract instrumentation or trauma can cause persistent hematuria. A history of prior treatment for bladder tumors or urolithiasis raises the possibility of recurrent disease. Renal papillary necrosis should be considered in patients with sickle-cell disease.

A history of significant cigarette smoking should be noted, as smokers have a two- to five-fold increased risk of developing transitional cell carcinoma (TCC) of the bladder. This risk decreases approximately 60% upon cessation of smoking, but remains elevated when compared with nonsmokers. Likewise, certain occupations with chemical exposure pose an increased risk for formation of TCC. Individuals at risk include dye workers (especially aniline, naphthylamine, and benzidine), automobile workers, chemical workers, rubber workers, dry cleaners, and painters.

A family history of nephrolithiasis, renal cystic disease, or bleeding disorder should prompt investigation for a corresponding inherited condition as the cause for the hematuria.

If tenderness and bruising are found over the ribs during the physical exam, a rib fracture and consequent renal injury may be present. Abdominal examination should assess for presence of a flank mass or bladder distention. In men, the genitalia should be examined for evidence of infection, and a prostate examination should assess gland size and consistency. In women, presence of urethral inflammation or prolapse should be noted, and a bimanual examination should evaluate the uterus, adnexae, and bladder. Lower extremity edema may indicate medical renal disease or lymphatic and vascular obstruction by a locally advanced malignancy.

A properly obtained mid-stream specimen is crucial for urinalysis. A catheterized specimen should be obtained from women who are menstruating or whose voided specimen contains numerous vaginal epithelial cells. Presence of proteinuria and RBC casts is highly suggestive of intrinsic renal disease. Presence of hematuria, pyuria, and bacteriuria indicates a urinary tract infection, which should be documented with a urine culture, and treated with an appropriate antimicrobial agent. Following resolution of the infection, a repeat urinalysis is performed. If the hematuria persists, urologic workup is indicated.

In patients with hematuria who are at increased risk for the development of recurrence of TCC, an additional urine specimen may be obtained for cytologic analysis. Cytologic criteria for malignancy include nuclear pleomorphism, prominent nucleoli, increased nuclear-to-cytoplasm ratio, and mitotic figures. Voided urine specimens as well as bladder barbitage (washing) specimens may be obtained for cytology. More exfoliated cells can be obtained for analysis by irrigating the bladder with saline. A positive voided urine cytology with a negative bladder barbitage cytology is suggestive of an upper tract source for the abnormal cells.

Urine cytology is 95% accurate for detecting high-grade TCC and CIS. However, the accuracy for detecting low-grade TCC is only 30–50%. The low accuracy of urine cytology for the detection of low-grade TCC has led to the development of additional urine tests as potential replacements or adjunct tests for urine cytology. These additional tests include the nuclear matrix protein test and the bladder tumor antigen test. Both tests demonstrate approximately 60% accuracy in detecting low-grade TCC. All urine screening tests have a significant false-negative rate for the detection of TCC. Therefore, all patients with hematuria must undergo definitive diagnostic evaluation regardless of the results of these tests.

The standard diagnostic evaluation for hematuria includes upper tract imaging followed by cystoscopy. If the patient's serum creatinine is normal, an intravenous pyelogram (IVP) is obtained. If the creatinine is elevated or if a contrast allergy is present, renal ultrasonography is performed. Renal masses, stones, and hydronephrosis are readily appreciated with either imaging modality. An IVP has the additional advantage of visualizing the ureters, which are poorly seen with ultrasound. If obstruction is present, delayed IVP films are obtained to quantify the degree of obstruction. Further upper tract imaging with CT scanning is indicated for renal parenchymal masses. Filling defects within the collecting system generally are evaluated next, with retrograde pyelography and ureteroscopy. Occasionally, a patient with hematuria has had a recent abdominal CT scan obtained for other reasons. If the CT was performed with intravenous contrast enhancement, and the upper tracts appear normal, no further upper tract imaging is necessary.

Examination of the lower urinary tract can be easily performed in the office setting with flexible cystoscopy. The urethra is rarely the source of bleeding in women, but urethroscopy may demonstrate inflamed urethral mucosa or a urethral tumor. In men, the anterior urethra may show signs of urethritis. Particular attention must be paid to the length, vascularity, and degree of visual obstruction within the prostatic urethra. On cystoscopy, the entire bladder must be examined for sources of bleeding such as tumors, stones, and erythematous patches suggestive of CIS. Bladder diverticuli must be thoroughly inspected, as tumors may be hidden within them. Occasionally, bloody efflux from a ureteral orifice may be seen, indicating an upper tract source for the bleeding. Following cystoscopy, a bladder barbitage may be obtained for cytologic analysis.

Cystoscopy should follow upper tract imaging so that upper tract abnormalities may be further evaluated with retrograde pyelograms and ureteroscopy, if necessary. If ultrasonography was performed, retrograde pyelograms must be obtained subsequently to visualize the ureter. These additional studies are carried out in the cystoscopy suite under an anesthetic.

In 5–10% of patients presenting with hematuria, no definite cause is found. Those with gross hematuria should be re-evaluated. Those with asymptomatic microscopic hematuria can be followed, as the likelihood of tumor development in these patients is less than 5%. However, a significant increase in the degree of hematuria or new onset of flank pain or voiding symptoms should prompt reevaluation.

The present patient had a significant smoking history and was therefore at increased risk for the development of TCC. Her negative urine cytology did not preclude further diagnostic workup. After the office cytoscopy, an IVP was obtained, which was normal. An outpatient transurethral resection of the lesion was performed under an anesthetic in the cystoscopy suite. Pathology revealed a low-grade, noninvasive transitional cell carcinoma.

Clinical Pearls

1. A urinalysis finding of greater than 3 RBC/hpf requires urologic evaluation.
2. The most common cause of gross hematuria in patients over the age of 50 is bladder cancer.
3. Cigarette smoking increases the risk of bladder cancer two- to fivefold.
4. In the adult male, terminal hematuria is most likely from a source in the prostate or at the bladder neck.
5. Persistent hematuria following successful treatment of a urinary tract infection requires urologic evaluation.
6. Urine cytology detects high-grade urothelial tumors and CIS, but may not detect a significant proportion of low-grade tumors.
7. A positive voided urine cytology with a negative bladder barbitage cytology is suggestive of an upper tract source for the abnormal cells.

REFERENCES

1. Mariani AJ, Mariani MC, Macchioni C, et al: The significance of adult hematuria: 1000 hematuria evaluations including risk-benefit and cost-effectiveness analysis. J Urol 141:350–355, 1989.
2. Murakami S, Igarashi T, Hara S, Shimazaki J: Strategies for asymptomatic microscopic hematuria: A prospective study of 1034 patients. J Urol 144:99–101, 1990.
3. Howard RS, Golin AL: Long-term followup of asymptomatic microhematuria. J Urol 145:335–336, 1991.
4. Mariani AJ: The evaluation of adult hematuria: A clinical update. AUA Update Series 17:186–192, 1998.

PATIENT 62

A 73-year-old man with urinary incontinence following radical prostatectomy

A 72-year-old man underwent a prostate needle biopsy due to an elevated prostate-specific antigen (PSA) of 10.6 with a normal digital rectal examination. The biopsy demonstrated Gleason's grade 4+3 prostate cancer in the right-sided cores. A staging bone scan was negative for metastatic disease, and the patient underwent a radical retropubic prostatectomy. He was potent preoperatively, and the left neurovascular bundle was spared. The pathology specimen showed Gleason's grade 4+3 adenocarcinoma involving approximately 25% of the total prostate volume, with no involvement of the capsule or lymph nodes, and negative surgical margins. The Foley catheter was removed 2 weeks postoperatively.

Since that time, he has had persistent leakage of urine, for which he wears a Cunningham clamp during the day and a condom catheter at night. He does not void due to the lack of bladder filling. He has not attempted intercourse because of the leakage. The leakage has persisted for 1 year despite the use of Kegel exercises. He now presents for further evaluation. His PSA has remained undetectable since surgery.

Physical Examination: General: upon standing, urine drips freely from the patient's urethral meatus. Vital signs: normal. Abdomen: soft, no masses or tenderness; well-healed lower midline surgical scar; bladder not palpable. Genitalia: phallus circumcised, no lesions, scrotum normal. Digital rectal examination: normal anal sphincter tone, empty prostatic fossa.

Laboratory Findings: CBC, serum electrolytes, BUN, creatinine, fasting blood sugar: normal. Urinalysis: 0–2 WBC/hpf, 0 RBC/hpf, no bacteria, rare epithelial cells. Urine culture: negative. Serum PSA: < 0.2 ng/dl.

Question: What is the single most important factor in preventing post-prostatectomy incontinence?

Answer: Surgical technique

Discussion: The surgical removal of the prostate, or prostatectomy, can be performed in a variety of ways, depending on the disease being treated, patient characteristics, and surgeon's experience. Surgery for symptomatic benign prostatic hyperplasia (BPH) involves removal of the obstructing adenoma (transition zone); the prostate capsule (peripheral zone) remains intact. This removal generally is accomplished via transurethral resection of the prostate (TURP), unless the prostate is quite large. Larger prostates are removed via open prostatectomy, by making an abdominal incision. The prostate can be approached either through the bladder (suprapubic prostatectomy) or beneath the pubis in the retropubic space (retropubic prostatectomy). Following either type of surgery for BPH, the patient remains at risk for the development of prostate cancer and must continue to be screened with a yearly PSA and digital rectal examination.

Surgery for prostate cancer involves removal of the entire prostate. This procedure, called radical prostatectomy, requires an anastomosis between the bladder neck and urethra. Radical prostatectomy can be performed through a retropubic approach or a perineal approach, depending on the surgeon's preference.

Urinary incontinence is an uncommon but devastating complication encountered after all types of prostatectomy. An understanding of the relevant anatomy and physiology of male urinary continence is critical to understanding the etiology, prevention, and treatment of this complication.

Urinary continence requires a stable bladder and a competent bladder neck/urethral sphincter mechanism. Incontinence due to an overactive bladder is termed urge incontinence, while incontinence due to a poorly functioning outlet is called stress incontinence. Urinary retention with intermittent leakage from an overdistended bladder is called overflow incontinence. In men, stress incontinence is exceedingly rare in the absence of neurologic disease or surgical insult.

The continence mechanism in the male has been arbitrarily divided into an internal sphincter and external sphincter. The **internal sphincter** is not a sphincter per se, but rather the combination of the bladder neck, prostate, and proximal urethral smooth muscle. This tissue is removed during all types of prostatectomy. The **external sphincter** is located distal to the prostate, at the membranous urethra. Endoscopically, it may be identified just distal to the verumontanum. The external sphincter consists of the compressible urethra mucosa, urethral smooth muscle, urethral striated muscle, and the levator ani musculature. Damage to these structures during prostatectomy results in stress urinary incontinence.

Incontinence following TURP or open prostatectomy is quite uncommon, with a reported incidence of 0.5–3%. During TURP, the verumontanum is used as a landmark, and resection distal to this structure is avoided. In patients with abnormal anatomy (due to locally advanced prostate cancer or prior radiation therapy) or neurologic pathology (e.g., Parkinson's disease, myasthenia gravis), the risk of incontinence is much higher. Patient's with prolonged bladder neck obstruction may have some degree of detrusor instability, resulting in postoperative urge incontinence. Incomplete resection or detrusor hypocontractility can lead to postoperative urinary retention and overflow incontinence.

The majority of men treated for post-prostatectomy incontinence have undergone radical prostatectomy. In fact, most patients are initially incontinent to some degree following this procedure. The symptoms usually resolve within several months; therefore, aggressive treatment is not warranted for at least 6 months postoperatively. The incidence of *persistent* incontinence varies widely depending on the study methodology and definitions of continence. Chart review analyses of modern series generally report an incidence of 5–10%, with severe incontinence in < 5% of patients. Patient questionnaire–based analyses indicate some degree of incontinence in over 50% of patients, and severe incontinence in 25%.

Surgical technique is critical in avoiding incontinence after radical prostatectomy. Intraoperative preservation of as much urethral length as possible is essential to preserve the external sphincter. A careful vesicourethral anastomosis is also important, as incontinence frequently is associated with anastomotic scarring or stricture. Nerve-sparing procedures have been associated with a lower rate of incontinence, but it is unclear whether this is due to a contribution to continence by the spared neurovascular bundles, or to more meticulous surgical technique. Incontinence almost invariably is accompanied by impotence, due to either associated intraoperative damage to the nerves or decreased libido on the patient's part. Patient characteristics are important, as younger men are less likely to be incontinent than older men, presumably due to less tissue strength and adaptability in the latter. Patients with shorter functional urethral lengths also may be at higher risk for incontinence.

The evaluation of all patients with post-prostatectomy incontinence should begin with a careful history and physical examination. Important components of the history include etiology, degree and duration of leakage, prior therapy, and current voiding symptoms. If the patient underwent a radical prostatectomy, current status of the prostate cancer (including most recent PSA level and adjuvant therapy) must be determined. The abdomen should be examined for a distended bladder, and the digital rectal examination should note evidence of recurrent disease. The genitalia and perineum should be examined for skin excoriation due to persistent dampness. Office cystoscopy often is useful to evaluate for an anastomotic stricture, bladder stone, bladder tumor, or retained suture which could be contributing to the patient's symptoms. If found, these complications should be treated and the patient should be reassessed subsequently. Video urodynamic studies should be obtained prior to any type of surgical therapy. These studies will further document the degree of incontinence, rule out bladder neck obstruction, confirm the presence of sphincteric deficiency, and document the presence of detrusor instability. Rarely, incontinence is found to be due to detrusor instability alone, which can be managed pharmacologically.

Treatment of post-prostatectomy incontinence depends on the duration and severity of the incontinence. Initially, reassurance and Kegel exercises are appropriate. Persistent incontinence must be evaluated to exclude the presence of urge incontinence or overflow incontinence. Mild stress incontinence may respond (rarely) to pharmacologic therapy with alpha-adrenergic agonists. The majority of patients, however, require surgical therapy. Currently accepted surgical treatments for male stress incontinence include the transurethral injection of collagen and placement of an **artificial urinary sphincter** (AUS). Collagen injections may be successful in those with mild degrees of leakage, but results have been disappointing in the majority of men despite numerous injections. Patients with severe leakage and those who have failed other measures are generally offered AUS placement. This treatment yields excellent long-term continence rates, but manual dexterity is required to operate the device. In addition, numerous revisions may be needed due to mechanical failure, urethral atrophy, urethral erosion, and infection. Patients who have received radiation therapy to the prostate are at particular risk for complications. A **bulbourethral sling** is an excellent alternative. It creates functionally significant elevation and compression of the bulbous urethra sufficient for dryness while allowing adequate urination. The initial reports indicate an 85% success rate in nonirradiated patients. Those who are not interested in surgical therapy for the incontinence may be managed with pads, diapers, condom catheters, and penile (Cunningham) clamps.

In the present patient, it is unlikely that the leakage will improve with observation, since his radical prostatectomy occurred a year ago. His PSA and digital rectal exam showed no evidence of disease recurrence. Cystoscopy showed no bladder neck contracture. Video urodynamics confirmed the presence of stress incontinence, with a low Valsalva leak point pressure of 50 cm H_2O, a normal bladder capacity, and no detrusor instability. Despite the severe degree of incontinence, he elected to undergo transurethral collagen injections. Three injections were performed, all of which caused temporary (1- to 2-week) improvement in the degree of leakage. He then underwent AUS placement, and now requires only one or two small pads per day for urinary leakage. He has soft erections, and is interested in therapy to improve them.

Clinical Pearls

1. The male continence mechanism consists of an internal urethral sphincter and an external urethral sphincter.

2. The internal sphincter is removed during all types of prostatectomy.

3. The external sphincter is located just distal to the verumontanum.

4. Surgical technique is the most important factor in preventing post-prostatectomy incontinence.

5. Following radical prostatectomy, continence may be regained up to 12 months postoperatively.

6. Video urodynamic testing should be obtained in all patients prior to surgical therapy for post-prostatectomy incontinence.

REFERENCES

1. Blaivas JG: Urinary incontinence after radical prostatectomy. Cancer suppl 75:1978–1982, 1995.
2. Gudziak MR, McGuire EJ, Gormley EA: Urodynamic assessment of urethral sphincter function in post-prostatectomy incontinence. J Urol 156:1131–1134, 1996.
3. Haab E, Yamaguchi R, Leach GE: Postprostatectomy incontinence. Urol Clin North Am 23:447–457, 1996.
4. Levy JA, Seay TM, Wein AJ: Postprostatectomy incontinence. AUA Update Series 15:58–68, 1996.
5. Schaeffer AJ, Clemens JQ, Ferari M, Stamey TA: The male bulbourethral sling procedure for post-prostatectomy incontinence. J Urol 159(5):1510–1515, 1998.

PATIENT 63

A 28-year-old man with azoospermia

A 28-year-old man presents for evaluation of infertility. He and his wife have been married for 3 years, and they have been trying for 2 years to achieve a pregnancy. Neither one has ever achieved a prior pregnancy. The patient has an unremarkable past medical and surgical history. He underwent normal sexual development, with puberty beginning at age 13. His wife is concurrently undergoing evaluation by her gynecologist.

Physical Examination: Vital signs: normal. General: healthy appearance. Head: normocephalic. Chest: normal breath sounds. Cardiac: normal. Abdomen: soft, nondistended, nontender, bowel sounds normal, no hernias. Genitourinary: normal, circumcised phallus; bilateral testes 25 ml volume, normal consistency; bilateral vasa deferentia and epididymides normal; no varicoceles; normal pubic hair distribution. Rectal: normal tone; prostate normal size, without masses.

Laboratory Findings:

	Volume (1.5–5.0 ml)	Density (> 60 million/ml)	Motility (> 60%)	Forward Progression (> 2)
Semen Analysis #1	0.5	0*	0	0
Semen Analysis #2	0.9	0*	0	0

* Semen pellet analysis after centrifugation revealed no spermatozoa.

Follicle-stimulating hormone (FSH) 9 (normal 4–10 mIU/ml); luteinizing hormone (LH) 7 (normal 6–9 mIU/ml); testosterone 340 (normal 200–1000 ng/dl); prolactin 8 (normal 3–20 ng/ml); semen fructose: negative.

Questions: What diagnostic study will help to confirm the diagnosis? What is the treatment of choice for this condition?

Diagnosis: Ejaculatory duct obstruction

Discussion: Fertility is the result of a complex interaction between the endocrine, neurological, and reproductive systems. Essential components in the male include testicular sperm production, sperm transport and maturation in the epididymis, and ejaculation. Failure of any one of these steps can result in azoospermia.

Infertility has received much attention over the last decade, due in part to the large number of people impacted by this problem as well as the significant advances in diagnosis and treatment. It is estimated that 85% of couples are able to achieve a pregnancy within 1 year of unprotected intercourse. Of the 15% of couples that cannot, approximately 30% are experiencing difficulty due to male factors alone, and another 20% are being hindered by a combination of male and female factors. Hence, an abnormal male factor is involved in about one half of infertile relationships.

In the past, an infertility evaluation typically was not initiated until after 12 months of unprotected intercourse. Physicians now recommend that couples obtain evaluations sooner, when they first identify the problem. By proceeding in this fashion, it is possible to minimize some of the anxiety and stress associated with waiting. Furthermore, for older couples, this quicker action makes use of valuable time in the race against the female partner's "biological clock." Due to educational and career demands, the current trend in the United States is to start a family later in life.

A thorough history is the foundation of the workup for male infertility. A number of factors must be considered. The age of the patient and his partner should be obtained, as well as information regarding any prior pregnancies by either one. Attention should be paid to the couple's sexual practices, including the use of lubricants. Several types of lubricant, including K-Y Jelly, Surgilube, saliva, and Keri Lotion, may impair sperm motility. The timing and frequency of intercourse should be examined. Sperm typically survive in the cervical mucus and cervical crypts for approximately 48 hours near the time of ovulation. Thus, intercourse with a frequency of every 2 days helps to maximize the odds of fertilization during the 12- to 24-hour period in which the egg is in transit within the fallopian tube.

Childhood and developmental history also are important aspects of the infertility evaluation. Cryptorchidism, or incomplete testicular descent, has an incidence of 3.4–5.8% in full-term boys. Fertility rates in couples in which the male has unilateral cryptorchidism average 81%, whereas the rates are only 50% if the male has a history of bilateral cryptorchidism. Patients should be asked about past pediatric surgical procedures, including pediatric herniorrhaphy, bladder neck surgery (Y-V plasty), and correction of testicular torsion, as each of these can be related to adult infertility. Childhood infections may be causative. A history of mumps, especially after the age of 11 or 12 (postpuberty), should be investigated. Mumps typically does not cause testicular insult in prepubescent males; however, when mumps infects postpubertal boys, approximately 30% develop unilateral and 10% develop bilateral mumps orchitis. The associated testicular damage can be severe, leading to impaired spermatogenesis and atrophy.

Regarding recent infections, any generalized illness (viral, bacterial, or febrile) can impair spermatogenesis, but the effects may not be evident in the semen for 1–3 months after the event. The spermatogenic process, including transit time in the ducts, takes approximately 3 months. Thus, an illness within the 3 months prior to the semen analysis should be kept in mind, and a followup semen analysis should be obtained at monthly intervals before final decisions regarding diagnosis and treatment are made.

Patients should be questioned about exposure to drugs and environmental toxins. Many drugs, such as tobacco, marijuana, alcohol, and cocaine, are believed to be detrimental to spermatogenesis. Environmental toxins, encountered both in the home and at the workplace, also can be damaging. The list of offensive items includes pesticides such as dibromochloropropane, heat, ionizing radiation, heavy metals, and some organic solvents. Early identification of the offending substances is important so that they can be removed from the patient's environment, hopefully minimizing any permanent injury that could result.

A thorough family history should be taken. Attention should be paid to a familial history of cystic fibrosis, which is associated with congenital bilateral absence of the vas deferens. Obviously, the presence of familial genetic or chromosomal abnormalities is important not only because of their impact on fertility, but also because of the importance of genetic counseling for these patients before initiating therapy.

The physical examination of patients presenting for infertility evaluation should be thorough, because any condition that impacts overall health can be detrimental to sperm production. A general inspection of the body should detect signs of inadequate virilization or androgen deficiency. These signs include eunuchoid body habitus, gynecomastia, and decreased body hair. The penis and scrotum should be carefully evaluated. Curvature of the phallus or ectopic location of the urethral meatus can result in abnormal deposition of the ejaculate within the vagina. Close attention should be paid to the scrotal exam, which should be done with the patient standing in a warm room. Testicular length, consistency, and volume (the latter is assessed with an orchidometer) should be determined. The normal testicular length is > 4 cm, and normal testis volume is > 20 ml. The presence of the epididymis should be confirmed. Cysts, induration, and other abnormalities should be noted. Finally, the scrotum should be evaluated for the presence of varicoceles. Extremely large varicoceles often are visible and have a characteristic "bag of worms" appearance. To examine for varicoceles, the patient should perform the Valsalva maneuver while the examiner palpates the spermatic cords. A detectable impulse usually is felt in patients with clinically apparent varicoceles. The impulse is due to transmission of the increased intra-abdominal pressure to the veins of the pampiniform plexus; this pressure impulse is typically not felt in normal patients. A Doppler stethoscope, which can be easily used in the clinic, and scrotal ultrasonography (to evaluate for veins > 3 mm and reversal of venous blood flow) can confirm clinically apparent varicoceles and detect those which are subclinical. Of note, venography rarely is used any more in the evaluation of these patients.

Laboratory testing is begun after the history and physical exam are completed. The tests ordered should be individually tailored to each patient. It is important to note that a semen analysis, although a vital component of the workup, is not a "fertility test." The interpretation should take into account crucial factors, such as how the specimen was collected and how it was analyzed. Semen collections should occur after an ejaculation abstinence period of 2–3 days, and they should be presented for analysis within 60–90 minutes of ejaculation. The specimen container should be wide-mouthed to ensure collection of the entire sample. The method of collection may be via masturbation, coitus interruptus, or condom collection (must be free of spermicidal agents). No one single semen analysis should be used to determine the patient's baseline. Usually 2–3 samples are collected and analyzed before a diagnosis and treatment plan are made. Semen parameters characteristically evaluated include: volume, density, motility, and forward progression. Normal values may vary slightly from lab to lab.

Several additional semen tests often are employed. An immunobead assay is done to detect the presence of antisperm antibodies, which can severely impair sperm motility. These antibodies may respond to treatment with corticosteroids. An assay for the presence of reactive oxygen species is important, for abnormally high concentrations can damage the sperm plasma membrane and impair its function. Reactive oxygen species are treated with vitamin E (antioxidant) therapy. The presence of genitourinary infections can be detrimental to sperm function as well. A microscopic examination of the semen alone is not sufficient to detect the presence of white blood cells (WBCs), because of the similarity between their appearance and the appearance of immature sperm. Therefore, a combination of semen culture and monoclonal antibody test to specifically detect the presence of seminal WBCs is necessary. Urethral swab cultures should be performed if there is a question of urethritis. Antimicrobial therapy is tailored appropriately, based on culture results.

Another common test is the Kruger Strict Morphology assay, which determines the percentage of normally shaped sperm within a sample, using standardized, rigid criteria. Normal values are > 4%. Values less than 4% are associated with impaired sperm function and reduced potential for successful fertilization. A number of tests are available to evaluate sperm function. However, in this age of extensive use of in vitro fertilization and intracytoplasmic sperm injection, whereby a sperm can be directly microinjected into an egg, many of the functional sperm problems associated with male factor infertility can be circumvented.

In addition to the semen analysis, hormonal testing usually is undertaken in the evaluation of the infertile male. Serum FSH should be measured prior to any intervention. Elevation of FSH two to three times above the normal value should be construed as an unfavorable sign associated with a probable primary testicular pathology. Many physicians only test LH and testosterone after obtaining an abnormal FSH result, as an isolated low LH or testosterone is relatively rare. Finally, a prolactin level should be ordered to rule out the presence of pituitary tumors impacting the hypothalamic-pituitary-testicular axis.

The appropriate treatment for the infertile couple depends on the patient's clinical problems, the age of the patient and his partner, and the desires of the couple.

In the present patient, the evaluation was begun with a history and physical examination, both of which were essentially normal. The workup continued with two semen analyses. Because of the findings of azoospermia, the semen sample was centrifuged and the resultant pellet examined under the microscope to rule out severe oligospermia. Both pellets were negative for sperm, thus confirming the diagnosis of azoospermia. At this point, with a normal FSH, LH, and testosterone, the differential diagnosis included: (1) failure of emission, (2) retrograde ejaculation, (3) an obstruction of the ejaculatory system, and (4) germinal cell failure.

Typically, failure of emission is seen in males with a history of testicular cancer who subsequently underwent retroperitoneal lymph node dissection (RPLND). Emission is primarily a function of the sympathetic nervous system. The dissection involved in an RPLND can result in damage to the sympathetic chain, which leads to impaired emission. These patients sometimes are treated effectively with sympathomimetic agents, such as ephedrine sulfate. Retrograde ejaculation generally is seen in a select subset of individuals, which includes patients who had RPLND, bladder neck, or pelvic surgery, as well as diabetics and those diagnosed with multiple sclerosis. In some of these patients, sympathomimetics can be helpful in facilitating bladder neck closure during emission and ejaculation, thus promoting antegrade ejaculation.

The next logical test for the present patient was a **semen fructose test**. The seminal vesicles produce fructose, which is delivered via the ejaculatory duct to the prostatic fossa with the rest of the seminal fluid during emission. Seminal fructose was absent, a finding highly suggestive of ejaculatory duct obstruction (EDO). The next appropriate test was **transrectal ultrasonography (TRUS)**, which is used to assess seminal vesicle diameter. *A diameter > 15 mm is suspicious for EDO*, and the seminal vesicle can be aspirated with a needle transrectally under ultrasound guidance. The presence of numerous sperm in the aspirate confirms obstruction, as seminal vesicle fluid normally contains no sperm. The patient had bilaterally dilated seminal vesicles, each measuring 19 mm in diameter. Subsequent seminal vesicle aspiration revealed numerous sperm present bilaterally, thus confirming the diagnosis of bilateral ejaculatory duct obstruction.

EDO may be congenital or may result from inflammation, ductal calculi, iatrogenic injury, and cysts. The treatment of choice is transurethral resection of the ejaculatory duct (TURED). This is performed cystoscopically with a cutting wire loop connected to electrocautery. The point of obstruction of the ejaculatory ducts is usually close to their point of termination within the prostatic urethra at the level of the verumontanum. Therefore, the verumontanum is resected, along with the underlying tissue. Our patient underwent TURED, with a return to normal semen volumes and sperm density and motility within 1 month. He and his wife conceived a child 4 months later.

Clinical Pearls

1. The ejaculatory ducts open in the majority of cases anterolateral to the orifice of the prostatic utricle.

2. Partial ejaculatory duct obstruction has been described, and semen analysis findings include oligospermia or azoospermia, decreased motility, and decreased ejaculate volume. In some men with only mild partial obstructions, semen parameters may approach normal.

3. In low-volume azoospermic patients in whom no ejaculatory duct obstruction is identified by fructose determinations or TRUS, a testis biopsy and touch preparation should be performed to rule out germinal cell failure.

4. Vasography (to evaluate for vasal obstruction) should be performed on those azoospermic patients with no evidence of EDO on fructose determination or TRUS and with normal testis biopsies.

5. Azoospermic patients with congenital unilateral absence of the vas deferens (CUAVD) should undergo renal ultrasonography to rule out renal agenesis, which has been reported in up to 80% of these men. The two often are concurrently absent due to their common embryologic origin. However, the incidence of such renal anomalies is much lower in CBAVD.

REFERENCES

1. Jarow JP: Evaluation and treatment of the azoospermic patient. Curr Prob Urol 2:4–30, 1992.
2. Goluboff EK, Stifelman ME, Fisch H: Ejaculatory duct obstruction in the infertile male. Urology 45:925–931, 1995.
3. Lipshultz LI, Howards SS: Infertility in the Male. St. Louis, Mosby-Year Book Inc., 1997.
4. Meacham RB, Lipshultz LI, Howards SS: Male infertility. In Gillenwater JY, Grayhack JT, Howards SS, Duckett JW (eds): Adult and Pediatric Urology, 3rd ed. St. Louis, MI, Mosby-Year Book, Inc., 1996, pp 1747–1802.
5. Orejuela E, Lipshultz LI: Effects of working environment on male reproductive health. Contemp Urol 10:86–92, 1998.

PATIENT 64

A 71-year-old man with overflow incontinence

A 71-year-old man presents to the emergency department with a complaint of an inability to urinate for the last 24 hours. Additional history reveals that the patient has experienced worsening symptoms of prostatism over the past 6 months. These symptoms include frequency, nocturia, urgency, and a weak urinary stream. He reports occasional urinary incontinence over the past 2 weeks. His past medical history includes mild hypertension and benign prostatic hypertrophy. He is currently treated for these conditions, by his primary medical doctor, with an alpha-blocker. Emergency personnel place a Foley catheter in the patient, and 1100 ml of clear urine is collected.

Physical Examination: Temperature 37.1°, pulse 84, respirations 22, blood pressure 180/95. General: appears fatigued and anxious. Abdomen: suprapubic region firm and distended. Genitalia: normal. Rectal: 40-gram firm prostate with no palpable nodules; stool negative for occult blood. Extremities: 2+ ankle edema.

Laboratory Findings: CBC normal; BUN 48 mg/dl; creatinine 2.4 mg/dl. Urine culture: negative. Prostate specific antigen drawn after rectal exam: 18.6 ng/ml (normal 4–10). Renal ultrasound: bilateral hydronephrosis.

Question: What are the workup and possible complications of this patient's urinary tract obstruction?

Diagnosis: Urinary tract obstruction secondary to benign prostatic hypertrophy

Discussion: Benign prostatic hyperplasia (BPH) is the most common benign tumor in men. Approximately 50% of men at age 60 have histologically identifiable prostatic hyperplasia. This increases to 90% by age 85 years. The incidence of bladder outlet obstruction secondary to prostatic hyperplasia also increases with age. At age 55 years, roughly 25% of men have obstructive voiding symptoms, and this increases linearly to approximately 50% by age 75 years. It has been estimated that a 40- to 50-year-old male has a 20–30% chance of requiring prostatectomy in his lifetime. Medical therapy can result in improvement of symptoms for many patients with BPH. However, dangerous complications of urinary obstruction from BPH, including acute urinary retention, urosepsis, or renal failure, occur in a small percentage of patients.

Acute urinary retention is the onset of a total inability to void. In some patients, urinary retention is the terminal event of steadily progressive urinary obstruction. Symptoms such as overflow incontinence worsen until the passage of urine is no longer possible. Surgical intervention typically is required for individuals with this disease course. In some patients, urinary retention develops more suddenly. These patients may be at various stages in the development of BPH. The episode of acute retention is often brought on by ingestion of alcohol, a prolonged delay in voiding, or the ingestion of anticholinergics, antidepressants, tranquilizers, or drugs with alpha-adrenergic activity such as over-the-counter cold medications. Many of these patients may respond to medical therapy and removal of the inciting agent.

BPH can cause what is termed extrinsic urinary tract obstruction. The obstruction is bilateral in relation to the kidneys and most often chronic. In addition to an expected irritative and obstructive voiding history, the physical complaints of patients with this condition may be rather nonspecific. Complaints may include: an increase in abdominal girth, ankle edema, hypertension, malaise, anorexia, headaches, weight gain, fatigue, and shortness of breath. In the setting of uremia, which some patients may develop, symptoms such as mental status changes, tremors, and gastrointestinal bleeding can occur. Laboratory data for patients with chronic bilateral obstruction also can be variable. Elevated BUN, creatinine, and urine sodium concentration are likely. Urine osmolality and urine-to-plasma creatinine ratio are generally decreased. Urinalysis may reveal hematuria, proteinuria, crystalluria, pyuria, and urinary casts. Obstruction coexisting with a bacterial urinary tract infection and/or fever should be considered a urologic emergency. The obstruction should be relieved promptly, the infection treated accordingly, and the patient observed closely for signs of systemic sepsis.

In addition to medical history, physical exam, and laboratory studies, a **baseline renal ultrasound** should be obtained as part of the workup for obstructive uropathy. Intravenous urograms (IVP) are generally not performed on these individuals due to the contraindication of the use of contrast in azotemic patients. Findings on ultrasound such as renal parenchymal thinning can give some indication as to the duration of obstruction. After the patient's obstruction is treated and resolves, subsequent renal ultrasonography can be used to evaluate if the patient's hydronephrosis resolves.

The initial treatment for BPH-induced urinary retention is placement of a Foley catheter or, if Foley catheterization is not possible, a suprapubic cystostomy tube. It is important to be aware that after placement of a Foley catheter, the patient's urine frequently becomes bloody. This common phenomenon is due to rapid refilling of the venous system with a possible rupture of a vein or veins lining the bladder mucosa. Often, emergency personnel clamp the Foley catheter after draining 500 cc of urine, to prevent this hematuria. Unfortunately, this curtailed catheterization does not allow complete decompression of the bladder and resolution of the obstruction. The urine generally clears on its own with the bladder decompressed by Foley catheterization.

After initial treatment of urinary tract obstruction with drainage, many patients are at risk for **postobstructive diuresis**. Patients who are most likely to develop a severe postobstructive diuresis are those who present with chronic obstruction, edema, congestive heart failure, hypertension, weight gain, azotemia, and, occasionally, uremic encephalopathy. The definition of postobstructive diuresis generally includes a urine output of greater than 3 L/day or a urine output greater than 200 ml/hr for 12–24 hours. The etiology for this polyuria and solute diuresis is most likely related to the patient's physiologic response to a volume-expanded state and inability to concentrate urine. There exist several hypotheses for the cause of postobstructive diuresis: (1) retained urea, sodium, and water during obstruction, (2) obstruction-induced impairment of the concentrating ability of the renal tubule, (3) an impaired ability to reabsorb sodium in the renal tubule, or (4) elevated hormones such as atrial natriuretic peptide.

The management and monitoring of the patient in the postobstructive period is critical. Resulting hyponatremia and hypokalemia can have hazardous neurologic and cardiac effects. If the patient's urine output meets the criteria for postobstructive diuresis, serum and urine electrolytes should be followed closely. Vital signs, including orthostatics, daily weight, and urine output, should be checked frequently. In most patients the diuresis will not persist, and BUN and creatinine levels return to normal within 24–48 hours. If the diuresis persists with low urine osmolality, the patient should receive intravenous fluid supplementation in addition to oral replacement. The accepted protocol calls for intravenous fluid replacement with 5% dextrose in 0.45% saline at a rate equal to half of the hourly urine output.

The bladder, as well as the kidney, undergoes obstruction-induced changes. Two types of obstruction-induced changes take place in the bladder. First, there are changes that lead to detrusor instability or decreased compliance, which can lead to symptoms of frequency and urgency. Second, more severe and chronic obstruction can lead to impaired detrusor contractility or even failure, possibly resulting in weakened urinary stream, hesitancy, intermittency, and increased retained urine. There is limited information on the natural history of human bladder musculature in the setting of chronic outflow obstruction. It is hypothesized that obstruction-induced changes in bladder wall contractility and cell-to-cell communication may result in bladder hypotonicity. There is further evidence that outflow obstruction may modulate neural-detrusor responses, resulting in bladder hypotonicity. Urodynamic assessment and pressure-flow studies of patients with prostatic obstruction should be done before surgical therapy is initiated. Pressure-flow studies also may be helpful in the evaluation of patients who have failed surgical treatment, to determine if the etiology of failure is bladder hypotonicity.

Surgical treatments for patients with severe BPH are numerous and rapidly evolving. Treatment must be tailored to the patient's age, surgical risk, glandular size, bladder function, and severity of symptoms. Several minimally invasive techniques are now available or currently under study for high-risk patients as well as geriatric patients.

The present patient has failed medical therapy and has strong evidence of chronic urinary obstruction due to BPH. He was encouraged to pursue surgical treatment options in light of the stage of his disease. A prostate ultrasound with needle biopsies was obtained to rule out malignancy and evaluate glandular mass. The patient's prostate mass was estimated at 40 grams, and biopsies were negative for adenocarcinoma of the prostate. The patient's age and relatively good health made him a good candidate for transurethral resection of the prostate (TURP). He subsequently underwent the procedure without complication, and can expect an 80–90% likelihood of symptomatic improvement.

Clinical Pearls

1. Benign prostatic hypertrophy is the most common benign tumor in men.

2. Severe BPH can cause extrinsic urinary tract obstruction leading to urinary retention, renal failure, and possibly sepsis.

3. Bladder drainage with Foley catheterization or suprapubic cystostomy is the immediate treatment of the patient in acute urinary retention.

4. Patients most likely to develop postobstructive diuresis are those who present with chronic obstruction, edema, congestive heart failure, hypertension, weight gain, or azotemia.

5. Chronic urinary obstruction due to BPH can induce changes in bladder detrusor function leading to bladder hypotonicity.

REFERENCES
1. Walsh PC, Retik AP, Stamey TA, Vaughan ED (eds): Campbell's Urology, 7th ed. Philadelphia, W.B. Saunders, 1998.
2. Gulmi FA, Felson D, Vaughan ED: Management of post-obstructive diuresis. AUA Update Series Lesson 23, Vol XVII, 1998.
3. Madsen FA, Bruskewitz RC: Clinical manifestations of benign prostatic hyperplasia, Urol Clin North Am 22(2):291–298, 1995.
4. Hollander JB, Diokno AC: Prostatism. Urol Clin North Am 23(1):75–85, 1996.

PATIENT 65

A 71-year-old man with urinary retention

A 71-year-old man presents to his primary care physician with the complaint of being unable to adequately empty his bladder for the preceding 24 hours. He has a history of an enlarged prostate, but his symptoms have been stable on a low dose of terazosin. He complains of malaise, but otherwise there is no history of fever, chills, dysuria, or flank pain. In addition, his past medical history consists of hypertension, for which he is taking diltiazem.

Physical Examination: Temperature 37.1°, pulse 76, blood pressure 176/92. General: moderate discomfort, otherwise healthy appearing. Abdomen: distended lower abdomen with suprapubic discomfort on palpation. Genitialia: circumcised phallus with a few nondescript, erythematous lesions of scrotum and left groin. Rectal: slightly decreased tone and decreased bulbocavernosus reflex; prostate moderately enlarged, nontender, without nodularity.

Laboratory Findings: CBC normal; creatinine 1.7 mg/dl. Foley catheter: 2 liters clear urine returned. Urinalysis: normal pH, trace leukocyte esterase, negative nitrites, 6–10 RBC/hpf, 0–5 WBC/hpf, no bacteria. Culture: negative.

Question: What are the possible causes of this patient's retention?

Diagnosis: Urinary retention secondary to herpes zoster

Discussion: Voiding dysfunction is one of the most common problems a urologist encounters. To address it, an understanding of the complex physiologic and pharmacologic interactions that occur with normal storage and emptying of urine is needed. In general, voiding dysfunction can be categorized based on whether these two actions are performed adequately: the problem is either a failure to store or a failure to empty urine. Some forms of dysfunction inevitably share impairment in both storage and emptying, and it is the general consensus that conversion to predominantly one or the other type of impairment with subsequent appropriate treatment provides the best results. This discussion primarily focuses on disorders related to failure to empty urine.

Whatever the cause, the initial management of acute failure to empty urine should be urinary catheterization. Catheterization usually is quick and easy, and it provides immediate relief of symptoms as well as prevents any of the pathologic sequelae related to urinary retention. If urinary catheterization proves difficult or impossible secondary to severe obstruction, suprapubic urinary diversion may be necessary. Once relief is obtained, the urine should be sent for urinalysis and urine culture to rule out infection as a cause. Routine serum chemistries should be performed to assess renal function and to look for any possible electrolyte disturbance. A thorough history and physical exam should then ensue, with close attention paid to the neurologic examination, specifically sensation, the bulbocavernosus reflex, and the deep tendon reflexes. Hypoactivity of these reflexes generally signifies a lower motor neuron lesion, whereas hyperactivity denotes an upper motor neuron lesion. The patient should be monitored for any sequelae to retention, such as postobstructive diuresis. Once these steps are taken, a thoughtful systematic and diagnostic approach can be undertaken to further classify the patient's problem into disorders of the bladder or disorders of the bladder outlet.

Disorders of the bladder proper include those associated with neurogenic, myogenic, psychogenic, or idiopathic causes. They may result from either temporary or permanent disruption in the normal mechanism needed for initiation and maintenance of detrusor contraction. This disruption is best demonstrated in so-called spinal "shock" following acute spinal cord injury. Herpes virus also can cause impaired sensation as well as disrupt the normal micturition reflexes by infecting the pelvic nerves. Myogenic causes include those circumstances where smooth muscle function is impaired,

as in severe infection or fibrosis. Inhibition of the normal micturition reflex can occur secondary to painful stimuli or it can be psychogenic in origin. **Disorders of the bladder outlet** generally can be attributed to anatomic outlet obstruction in men, such as that seen with benign prostatic hyperplasia. Urethral stricture disease and bladder neck contracture from prior surgery also are common causes of anatomic obstruction. Functional obstruction can occur at either the smooth or striated sphincter (dyssynergia) during micturition and is a common cause of voiding dysfunction in those patients with spinal cord injury.

Radiologic evaluation is often nonspecific, but may show patterns consistent with certain types of voiding dysfunction. For instance, cystography may reveal trabeculation, cellules, or diverticula; all would be consistent with obstruction. Endoscopic evaluation is often wise to rule out neoplasm as a cause for irritative or obstructive voiding symptoms, plus it aids in the diagnosis of anatomic outlet obstruction. Note, however, that endoscopic evaluation is not always consistent with urodynamic findings, and that clinical judgment always should guide decision making.

Urodynamics and video urodynamics have become very popular in recent years as interest in the physiology of voiding grows. Urine flowmetry is simple to perform, but does not distinguish between outlet obstruction and decreased detrusor contractility. Moreover, low urinary flow rates might be recorded in the context of low bladder volumes, and decreased bladder compliance may be misinterpreted as a failure to empty. Cystometry is more helpful in that it provides information on bladder compliance, sensation, and detrusor contractility. Video urodynamics involves simultaneous measurement of flow, detrusor pressure, and abdominal pressure coupled with fluoroscopic visualization of the micturition process. High voiding pressures (greater than 60 centimeters of water) and low urine flow rates (less than 10–12 cubic centimeters per second) are associated with obstruction. In addition, the site of obstruction may be elucidated on these studies, such as in cases of detrusor striated sphincter dyssynergia seen in spinal cord patients.

Therapy of bladder emptying disorders is aimed at either increasing intravesical (voiding) pressures or decreasing outlet resistance, depending on the particular problem. The simplest way to increase intravesical pressures is by using the Valsalva maneuver or external compression (Crede). These methods can be very efficient in emptying the bladder in appropriate patients, but obviously are difficult in the setting of severe spinal cord injury. Pharmacologic therapy exists for increasing detrusor contraction, though it has not been shown to be extremely effective. Acetylcholine is the primary neurotransmitter involved in detrusor contraction. Acetylcholine-like drugs are available (bethanechol) and are widely used, but there is no definitive, reproducible data to date to support their use. Alpha-adrenergic blockers have been tried in the hopes of removing the normal inhibitory role that the sympathetic nervous system plays in the micturition reflex. However, it is difficult to discern in these studies whether this is a real effect or if improvement results from decreasing outlet resistance. There is no effective surgical treatment for increasing bladder contractility.

In contrast, decreasing outlet resistance often involves surgical intervention. Transurethral resection remains the gold standard for relief of anatomic obstruction due to an enlarged prostate. A trial of medical therapy with alpha blockade should be offered. It is thought that the symptomatic improvement seen in benign prostatic hypertrophy with use of alpha blockers is due to reduction in stromal smooth muscle tone, thereby decreasing the dynamic component of outlet resistance. Dilation of urethral strictures is sometimes necessary to relieve obstruction. If the increased resistance is at the level of the bladder neck or smooth sphincter, alpha blockade is also useful. In extreme circumstances, surgical incision or reconstruction of the bladder neck may be necessary. If the obstruction is at the level of the striated sphincter, such as that seen with dyssynergia, then treatment with skeletal muscle relaxants has proved useful. The benzodiazepines and baclofen work through centrally mediated pathways. Dantrolene has a direct effect on skeletal muscle by interfering with excitation-contraction coupling. It is not used very much because of the tendency to induce profound generalized muscle weakness. Fatal hepatitis also has been reported in patients taking the medication for longer than 60 days, which limits its usefulness. When all else fails, clean intermittent catheterization may be necessary.

In the present patient, a careful review of the history revealed a remote incidence of herpes zoster. After admission, his scrotal and groin lesions flowered into fulminant herpetic vesicular lesions. He responded nicely to treatment with acyclovir and urinary catheter drainage, and upon removal of the catheter his voiding returned to baseline.

Clinical Pearls

1. Endoscopic findings during evaluation of voiding dysfunction may vary significantly from urodynamic findings.

2. Conversion to a single type of voiding disorder with subsequent treatment aimed at that type is recommended when dealing with mixed etiologies.

3. A thorough neurologic evaluation should be performed on anyone with urinary retention, rather than writing the disorder off as benign prostatic hypertrophy.

4. Alpha blocker therapy is useful not only in treatment of benign prostatic hypertrophy, but also in disorders of the bladder neck smooth musculature.

5. Video urodynamics can prove extremely helpful in the patient with a complicated history or suspected neurogenic origin of voiding dysfunction.

REFERENCES

1. Wein AJ: Pharmacological therapy. In Krane RJ, Siroky MB (eds): Clinical Neuro Urology. Boston, Little, Brown, 1991, pp 523–558.
2. Wein AJ: Drug therapy for neurogenic and non-neurogenic bladder dysfunction. In Seidmon EJ, Hanno PM (eds): Current Urologic Therapy, 3rd ed. Philadelphia, W.B. Saunders, 1994, pp 291–299.
3. Steers WD, Barrett DM, Wein AJ: Voiding function and dysfunction. In Gillenwater JY, Grayhack JT, Howards SS, Duckett JW (eds): Adult and Pediatric Urology, 3rd ed. St. Louis, Mosby, 1996, pp 1220–1326.

PATIENT 66

A 71-year-old man with azotemia

A 71-year-old man presents to the emergency department with a 3-day history of malaise and decreased urinary output. He denies any history of flank pain, hematuria, or antecedent voiding symptoms. There is no history of fever, nausea, or vomiting, although his appetite is somewhat decreased. He is an otherwise healthy gentleman, with the exception of some mild arthritis for which he occasionally takes ibuprofen. He has no known medical allergies.

The patient recently was given a prescription for amoxicillin after being diagnosed with sinusitis. He has been on the medication for the 3 days prior to presentation, but has not noticed a rash or any other ill effects of the medicine (see table).

Physical Examination: Temperature 37.4°, pulse 98, respirations 18, blood pressure 154/82. General: appears fatigued, no significant distress. Chest: clear. Cardiac: regular rhythm, no murmurs. Abdomen: soft, nontender, no masses. Genitourinary: no lesions, masses, or tenderness. Rectal: smooth, nonenlarged prostate.

Laboratory Findings: CBC: normal. BUN 54 mg/dl, creatinine 3.5 mg/dl. Potassium 6 mEq/L. Other electrolytes and liver function tests: normal. Urinalysis: 2+ proteinuria, 11–50 WBC/hpf with casts, 6–10 RBC/hpf. Urine osmolality: 250 mOsm/L.

Question: What is the significance of the laboratory values?

Diseases of the Tubulointerstitium Associated with Acute Intrinsic Renal Azotemia

Drug-Induced Allergic Interstitial Nephritis					Infections
β-Lactams	Other Antibiotics	NSAIDs	Diuretics	Other	
Ampicillin	Ethambutol	Aspirin	Chlorthalidone	α-Methyldopa	Bacterial
Amoxicillin	p-Aminosalicylate	Diflunisal	Furosemide	Allopurinol	Acute pyelonephritis*
Carbenicillin	Rifampin	Fenoprofen	Thiazides	Azathioprine	Leptospirosis
Methicillin	Sulfonamides	Glafenine	Ticrynafen	Carbamazepine	Scarlet fever
Nafcillin	Trimethoprim-	Ibuprofen		Cimetidine	Typhoid fever
Oxacillin	sulfamethoxazole	Idomethacin		Clofibrate	Legionnaire disease
Penicillin G	Ciprofloxacin	Meclofenamate		Diphenylhydantoin	Viral
Cephalexin		Mefenamic acid		Interferon alfa	Cytomegalovirus infection
Cephalothin		Naproxen		Phenindione	Measles
Cephradine		Phenazone		Phenobarbital	Infectious mononucleosis
Cefotaxime		Phenylbutazone		Phenylpropanolamine	Rocky Mountain spotted
		Tolmetin		Sulfinpyrazone	fever
					Other
					Candidiasis, other fungi†
					Toxoplasmosis

* Rare to get ARF unless bilateral disease in diabetic patients.

† May cause ARF by obstruction of tubules (fungus balls), in addition to causing acute interstitial nephritis.

Adapted from Brezis M, Rosen S, Epstein F: Acute renal failure. In Brenner BM, Rector FC Jr (eds): The Kidney, 5th ed. Philadelphia, WB Saunders, 1996, with permission.

Diagnosis: Acute renal failure secondary to drug-induced tubulointerstitial nephritis

Discussion: Acute renal failure (ARF) denotes an abrupt decline in renal function such that the normal homeostatic mechanisms of the kidney are impaired. ARF is a comprehensive term encompassing many etiologies, diagnoses, and pathophysiologic mechanisms. In the broadest sense, ARF can be divided into prerenal, renal (intrinsic), and postrenal causes. Prerenal failure results from inadequate perfusion of the kidneys, usually secondary to volume depletion, but not infrequently due to inadequate cardiac output as seen in congestive heart failure. Postrenal failure is invariably due to urinary tract obstruction, either anatomic or functional. Note that *both* kidneys must be involved, for unilateral obstruction with a functional contralateral kidney does not result in the degree of azotemia seen in ARF. Intrinsic renal failure has a variety of causes which, to one degree or another, impact on intrarenal vascular, glomerular, tubular, or interstitial function. The end result, however, is impairment in the biochemical processes of the kidney that maintain homeostasis.

ARF can be divided into **oliguric** (urine output less than 400 milliliters over 24 hours) or **nonoliguric** (urine output greater than 400 milliliters over 24 hours) types. Morbidity and prognosis is largely dependent on which category applies to the patient. Patients with nonoliguric renal failure have lower mortality rates (10–25% versus 50%), shorter hospital stays, and less chance of requiring dialysis when compared to those with oliguric ARF. In addition, the specific cause of the renal failure also impacts on recovery of renal function. Those with acute cortical necrosis or thrombotic phenomenon (thrombotic thrombocytopenic purpura or hemolytic uremic syndrome) have a greater than 65% chance of requiring dialysis. In contrast, those with acute tubular necrosis or interstitial nephritis have a better than 60% chance for recovery of fully normal renal function.

There are several diagnostic considerations that can aid in assignment of a particular patient to one of the aforementioned categories of ARF. Early recognition and assignment is important, not only for prognostic implications, but also to guide therapy so as to avoid conversion from nonoliguric failure to oliguric failure—or even frank anuria. Initial workup should include a thorough history and physical examination. Any recent intake of possible offending agents should be noted. Examination should be geared towards assessing the patient's overall fluid status as well as any outward signs of electrolyte disturbance. Serum BUN and creatinine as well as serum electrolytes should be obtained. A BUN/creatinine ratio greater than 10:1

is highly suggestive of a prerenal cause. Urine also should be obtained for urinalysis, urine osmolality, and urine chemistries. Frequently, intrinsic renal failure manifests with tubular epithelial casts or RBC casts. Postrenal failure may show free RBCs, malignant cells, or crystal formation. Urine sodium concentration is usually less than 15 mEq/L and urine osmolality greater than 450 mOsm/L in prerenal failure, due to the kidney's retained ability to avidly reabsorb filtered sodium and water in response to volume depletion. In contrast, urine sodium is greater than 40 mEq/L and osmolality less than 300 mOsm/L in intrinsic ARF, which reflects the inability to reabsorb sodium and adequately concentrate urine due to tubular and interstitial damage.

Alterations in potassium and hydrogen ion excretion are common in intrinsic ARF, resulting in a hyperkalemic metabolic acidosis. An electrocardiogram should be obtained, if warranted, and these electrolyte disturbances corrected accordingly. The administration of sodium polystyrene, a resin that binds potassium in the gut, is often helpful, as is the simultaneous administration of glucose and insulin if the hyperkalemia is severe. Often, the severity of total body potassium overload may be underestimated due to a concurrent acidosis, which results in a shift of potassium intracellularly. This shift should be factored into the treatment regimen. If postrenal failure is suspected, a renal ultrasound and catheterization should be performed, as catheterization can prove therapeutic as well as diagnostic.

The pathophysiology of **prerenal azotemia** relates to a reduction in renal blood flow and decreased efferent arteriolar pressure, which cause decreased filtration of renal plasma. Decreased filtration greatly increases the reabsorption of solutes by the renal tubular system. Urea is reabsorbed in large amounts, and what little creatinine is excreted cannot be reabsorbed, which results in the increased BUN/creatinine ratio in serum. Treatment of prerenal failure is aimed at the underlying primary disease, and usually consists of volume repletion or improvement in myocardial function to effect greater renal blood flow.

Postrenal failure also causes a reduction in renal blood flow and glomerular filtration rate (GFR) by causing increased hydrostatic pressure throughout the entire nephron. Destruction of tight junctions in the tubules occurs, causing increased permeability and decreased net sodium and water reabsorption. Renin, prostaglandins, and thromboxane have been studied in obstructive uropathy, but their roles are not completely understood. After the obstruction is relieved, concentrating ability often remains impaired, resulting in large volumes of urine and sodium losses—the so-called postobstructive diuresis. Timing of the return of concentrating ability is variable and relates to the acuteness of the obstruction as well as the degree of washout of the medullary interstitium. Obviously, treatment is directed at the site of obstruction. Urethral catheters are the mainstay of therapy, but suprapubic and even percutaneous nephrostomy drainage are occasionally necessary.

Intrinsic renal failure is most commonly due to either acute tubular necrosis (ATN) or acute interstitial nephritis (AIN). ATN is usually a result of ischemic injury, such as that seen in hemorrhagic shock, aortic cross-clamping in trauma or vascular surgery, or renovascular clamping during nephron-sparing surgery. Direct nephrotoxic tubular damage also can occur with drugs (aminoglycosides), myoglobin (crush injuries), and administration of intravenous contrast agents. The proposed mechanisms of intrinsic ARF include vasomotor changes, increased tubule permeability, tubular obstruction, and decreased ultrafiltration. All of these have some merit; realistically, intrinsic ARF is likely multifactorial.

AIN is also characterized by a decreased GFR, and it is usually associated with some degree of proteinuria as well as an active urinary sediment. Eosinophiluria and, less commonly, eosinophilia may be present. Tubular dysfunction is the rule, and may manifest as various electrolyte disturbances as well as concentrating defects. AIN can be divided into drug-related, infection-related, and idiopathic causes. Semi-synthetic penicillins, sulfa drugs, nonsteroidal antiinflammatory drugs, and histamine-2 blockers all have been implicated. AIN is becoming more common with the widespread use of such agents. AIN also has been associated with viral infections (cytomegalovirus, Epstein-Barr virus), as well as various bacterial infections such as leptospirosis, diphtheria, and toxoplasmosis. Treatment of intrinsic renal failure is directed at supportive therapy and correction of accompanying electrolyte abnormalities. In the case of AIN, the offending agent should be withdrawn.

In the present patient, the BUN/creatinine ratio, the RBC casts on urinalysis, and the urine osmolality suggested intrinsic ARF. Ingestion of a semi-synthetic penicillin, amoxicillin, pointed to drug-related acute interstitial nephritis. He responded to withdrawal of the amoxicillin and conservative supportive therapy. His renal function returned to baseline within 2 weeks, and he suffered no significant sequelae.

Clinical Pearls

1. Early recognition and assignment to prerenal, intrinsic, or postrenal causes has a profound impact on the outcome of ARF.

2. Urine osmolality and chemistries provide a fast, easy way to classify ARF.

3. The degree of hyperkalemia may be understated in ARF due to a coexisting metabolic acidosis.

4. The concentrating defects associated with urinary obstruction may linger for several days to weeks after the obstruction is relieved and the creatinine normalizes.

5. Eosinophils in the urine may signify a drug-induced interstitial nephritis, and a thoughtful search for an offending agent should ensue.

REFERENCES

1. Palter MS: Drug-induced nephropathies. Med Clin North Am 74(4):909–917, 1990.
2. McDougal WS: Kidney. In Gillenwater JY, Grayhack JT, Howards SS, Duckett JW (eds): Adult and Pediatric Urology, 3rd ed. St. Louis, Mosby, 1996, pp 617–642.
3. Bennett WM: Drug nephrotoxicity: An overview. Renal Failure 19(2):221–224, 1997.

PATIENT 67

A 52-year-old man with history of gout presenting with acute renal colic

A 52-year-old man presents with a 24-hour history of acute-onset right flank pain initially followed by intermittent gross hematuria. The pain radiates to the right groin. He denies fevers, chills, and arthralgias. He does complain of some increase in urinary frequency, but otherwise denies dysuria or decreased urine output. He has a history of gout and takes colchicine and nonsteroidal anti-inflammatories during flare-ups of his disease. His last acute episode was approximately 9 months ago. He currently denies symptoms of acute gout. He has a history of hypercholesterolemia and is on simvastatin. He has no known allergies. There is no family history of kidney or bladder problems. He denies any prior episodes of flank pain or hematuria.

Physical Examination: Temperature 37.5°, pulse 88, respirations 16, blood pressure 141/72. General: healthy appearing, mild distress secondary to pain. Chest: clear. Cardiac: regular rhythm, no murmurs. Abdomen: slightly obese, mild right flank pain to deep palpation only, no costovertebral tenderness elicited. Genitourinary: no lesions, masses, or tenderness. Rectal: smooth, nonenlarged prostate.

Laboratory Findings: WBC 11,500/μl. BUN 21 mg/dl, creatinine 1.4 mg/dl. Electrolytes: normal. Serum calcium 10.7 mg/dl, uric acid 10 mg/dl. Urinalysis: pH 5, positive nitrites, > 100 RBC/hpf, 6–10 WBC/hpf, 1+ bacteria. Urine culture: sterile. Abdominal x-ray: negative. Intravenous pyelogram and noncontrast CT scan: see figures.

Questions: What are the metabolic and pathologic consequences of his disorder? What are the mainstays of therapy?

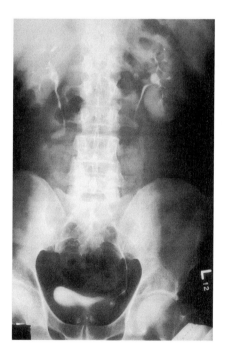

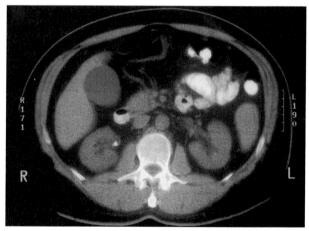

Diagnosis: Uric acid lithiasis

Discussion: Uric acid calculi account for less than 10% of all urinary stones in the United States. This incidence is somewhat higher in certain parts of the globe, namely some Middle Eastern countries; the reason is not exactly clear, but climates as well as genetic factors possibly play a role. The only mammals prone to forming uric acid calculi are humans and the Dalmatian coach hound. In most mammals, uric acid, which is a major end product of purine metabolism, is broken down by the hepatic enzyme uricase into a more water-soluble form (uric acid is insoluble in water). Humans lack this enzyme. The Dalmatian possesses this enzyme, but excretes large amounts of uric acid into the urine due to lack of proximal tubular reabsorption.

Under normal metabolic conditions, uric acid is filtered by the glomeruli, but is readily absorbed by the proximal tubular epithelium. Instead of being recirculated and broken down further in the liver, the uric acid then is actively secreted by the distal tubule. It is destined to exist in one of two forms: a nonionized form that is very insoluble, or as a urate salt, which is approximately 20 times more soluble than its nonionized counterpart. The proportion of uric acid that exists in the insoluble form is a function of the pKa of uric acid and the pH of the urine in which it resides. The pKa of uric acid is approximately 5.5. This means that at a pH of 5.5, exactly half of the uric acid exists in the insoluble nonionized form. While humans normally excrete a urine that is acidic with respect to serum (normal urinary pH 6–7), this is well above the pKa of uric acid such that supersaturation and crystal formation does not occur. As the urine becomes more and more acidic, more of the uric acid exists in an insoluble form, and crystallization occurs. At a urinary pH of 5, for instance, urinary precipitation occurs with only 60 milligrams of uric acid per liter of urine. The average human excretes approximately 400 milligrams of uric acid each day, so a urine pH of 5 would require over 6 liters of urine output each day to avoid crystallization! Likewise, at a pH of 6, urinary saturation does not occur until the urine contains 220 milligrams of uric acid per liter. The remaining ionized urate reacts with both potassium and sodium to form urate salts. Potassium urate is much more soluble than sodium urate, so increasing sodium concentration in the urine actually makes dissolution less likely, and increasing potassium excretion favors dissolution.

Other factors also have an impact on stone formation. Postprandial elevations in urinary pH have been demonstrated in normal individuals. There is some evidence that people prone to forming uric acid stones fail to alkalinize their urine. Low urinary volumes certainly play a role in supersaturation, and people who excrete low volumes of acidic urine are at higher risk. Such individuals include patients with severe inflammatory bowel disease or with ileostomies that bypass the normal colonic water and bicarbonate reabsorption mechanisms.

Uric acid lithiasis can be divided into four broad categories. In the first category are diseases associated with elevations in serum uric acid, including primary gout and other metabolic diseases such as Lesch-Nyhan syndrome. About one quarter of patients with gout form uric acid stones, and approximately one quarter of patients with uric acid stones have gout at some time. Patients with increased cell turnover rates (e.g., those with myeloproliferative disorders or receiving chemotherapy) are also prone to hyperuricemia, due to the purines released from cell breakdown. The second category comprises those patients with a predilection for dehydration (e.g., patients at risk for chronic diarrhea, ulcerative colitis, severe radiation proctocolitis, or with ileostomies). The third category encompasses patients with hyperuricosuria without elevated serum levels of uric acid. Hyperuricosuria is defined as output of greater than 800 milligrams a day in men and greater than 750 milligrams a day in women. Certain medications, namely thiazide diuretics, cause increased excretion of uric acid and may lead to stone formation. The fourth and final category consists of people who form stones despite normal serum levels of uric acid and no demonstrable hyperuricosuria. These people typically have a persistently acidic urine. This condition is defined as idiopathic uric acid lithiasis.

Uric acid stones usually present with symptoms of typical renal colic. Pure uric acid stones are radiolucent on plain films. However, the presence of a calcium shell or a very large stone may cause some opacification. Uric acid stones appear as radiolucent filling defects on intravenous and retrograde pyelograms; therefore, the differential must include tumor, blood clot, and sloughed renal papilla. Computed tomography has become popular of late in the workup of patients with suspected urolithiasis. A density in the urinary tract that is less intense than bone or typical calcium stones is consistent with uric acid calculi in the proper clinical setting. Thus CT scans can prove helpful in the absence of calcification on plain films. The combination of typical renal colic, acidic urine, and radiographic evidence makes the diagnosis of uric acid stones a reasonably straightforward one.

Treatment of uric acid calculi should consist of a conservative approach centered on increasing urinary volumes and urinary alkalinization. All patients with presumed uric acid stones deserve an initial conservative approach unless earlier operative intervention is absolutely necessary. Surgical intervention is reserved for those who fail medical therapy. Patients should be encouraged to drink a large amount of fluids (at least 64 ounces a day), with a goal of 3 liters of urine output per day. Urinary alkalinization can be achieved in a variety of ways. Sodium bicarbonate can be given at a dose of 50 to 100 mEq per day, and this is quite inexpensive. Urine pH should be followed with a target pH of 7.0–7.5. Alternatively, potassium citrate can be administered in 15 mEq doses three to four times daily. This is the preferred method in those with normal renal function because potassium urate is more soluble than sodium salt. Intravenous alkalinization is sometimes necessary, especially in those patients who cannot tolerate the oral preparations. Caution should be exercised to avoid making the urine too alkaline, as this may cause precipitation of calcium phosphate stones.

For those with hyperuricemia, a diet low in purine-rich foods such as red meats and chicken is recommended. In addition, allupurinol should be considered. Allopurinol is a xanthine oxidase inhibitor that blocks the formation of uric acid during purine metabolism.

Finally, if all else fails, standard techniques can be employed to render a patient stone free. These techniques include endoscopic stone manipulation and extracorporeal lithotripsy. These stones are usually of mixed uric acid and calcium components, which is why they may not have responded to conservative measures.

In the present patient, a stone is not visible on plain radiographic imaging. There is a filling defect, however, on the intravenous pyelogram, and a stone is visible on CT imaging. This, in association with the low urinary pH, is consistent with a uric acid stone. This patient failed a trial of medical management, and subsequently underwent retrograde endoscopic extraction of his stone, without incident.

Clinical Pearls

1. Uric acid stones account for less than 10% of all stones in the United States.

2. It is extremely rare for uric acid stones to form in a urine pH greater than 6.5.

3. Although *most* uric acid stones are radiolucent, large stones or those with a calcium shell may be faintly visible on plain films.

4. Therapeutic goals include a urinary volume of at least 3 liters a day and a urinary pH of 7–7.5.

5. Overalkalinization of the urine may cause formation of calcium phosphate stones and should be avoided.

REFERENCES

1. Gutman AB, Yu TF: Uric acid nephrolithiasis. Am J Med 45:756–799, 1968.
2. Hess B: Prophylaxis of uric acid and cystine stones. Urol Res 18:541, 1990.
3. Jenkins AD: Calculus formation. In Gillenwater JY, Grayhack JT, Howards SS, Duckett JW (eds): Adult and Pediatric Urology, 3rd ed. St. Louis, Mosby, 1996, pp 461–506.

PATIENT 68

A 21-year-old woman with left flank pain

A 21-year-old woman without significant past medical history presents with left flank pain. She denies any fevers, chills, hematuria, or previous similar complaints. Her pain radiates from her left side to the left inguinal region episodically. She states that her two brothers and her mother have a history of kidney stones.

Physical Examination: Temperature 37.2°, pulse 85, respirations 18, blood pressure 150/80. General: healthy appearance. Abdomen: benign, no masses palpated. Back: mild left costovertebral tenderness. Genitalia: normal, no hernias. Pelvic/rectal: normal.

Laboratory Findings: Urinalysis: 0–5 WBC/hpf, 11–50 RBC/hpf, pH 5.5. Urine culture: negative. WBC 11,100/µl, hemoglobin and platelet counts normal. BUN 7 mg/dl, creatinine 0.6 mg/dl. Serum uric acid, calcium, and phosphorus: normal. Fresh, first morning void: hexagonal crystals on microscopic examination (see figure). Intravenous pyelogram: mild left hydronephrosis; 9-mm radiopaque stone in left ureteropelvic junction; 5-mm radiopaque stone in lower pole of left kidney; nonobstructing 4-mm radiopaque stone in lower pole of right kidney.

Question: What is the probable diagnosis?

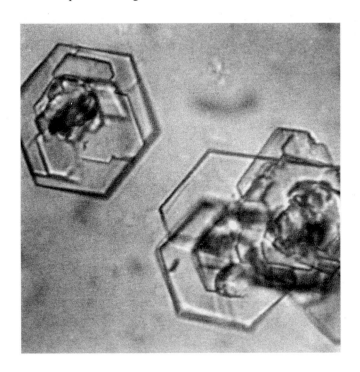

Diagnosis: Cystinuria with resultant urolithiasis

Discussion: Cystine stones account for 1–2% of all urinary calculi overall. Cystinuria is an autosomal recessive disorder of transmembrane transport resulting in defective absorption in the intestines and resorption in the proximal tubule of the dibasic amino acids (cystine, ornithine, lysine, and arginine). The gene responsible for cystinuria has been located to chromosome 2p. Homozygous expression of cystinuria has a prevalence of 1:20,000, and the heterozygous expression is 1:20 to 1:2000. Cystine lithiasis is the only clinical manifestation of cystinuria and only occurs in homozygotes. Stones can occur in childhood, but the peak incidence of cystine stones is in the second to third decade of life.

Cystine stones are moderately radiopaque and grossly appear to be yellowish and waxy. The radiopacity is secondary to the disulfide bond between the two cysteine molecules that form cystine. Cystine often forms multiple stones that can be large in size and may form staghorn calculi. It is poorly soluble at normal urinary pH, and **solubility is pH dependent**. The pKa is 8.3. Cystine solubility rises exponentially as pH rises: at a pH of 5, the solubility of cystine is 300 mg/L; at a pH of 7, the solubility is 400 mg/L; and at a pH of 8, the solubility is 1000 mg/L.

The diagnosis of cystinuria can be made by identifying the typical hexagonal crystals on a fresh, first morning urine specimen, or by detecting a magenta ring produced by the cyanide-nitroprusside calorimetric test. This test is positive for urinary cystine levels greater than 75 mg/L. If the screening cyanide-nitroprusside test is positive, urinary cystine excretion should be quantitated with amino acid chromatography; more than 250 mg of cystine over 24 hours is diagnostic of cystinuria. Urinary excretion is less than 30 mg per day in healthy adults, 100–400 mg per day in heterozygotes, and greater than 400 mg per day in homozygotes.

The goal of therapy is to lower cystine concentration in urine to less than 200 mg/L. Methionine is the metabolic precursor of cystine, and low methionine diets are theoretically beneficial; however, they are pragmatically unpalatable, leading to poor compliance. Decreasing sodium intake may decrease cystine excretion, as the presence of sodium increases cystine excretion, but the results are thought to be modest at best.

Oral hydration (up to 4 L per day) with urinary output of up to 3 L per day has been effective in preventing urolithiasis in two-thirds of stone-forming cystinuric patients. Alkalinization of urine to a pH greater than 7.5 is necessary because the pKa of cystine is 8.3. Potassium citrate (15–20 mEq two to three times per day) is the most commonly used oral alkalinizing agent. Sodium bicarbonate (15–25 g per day) is sometimes used. Acetazolamide (250 mg three times per day) increases urinary bicarbonate excretion by inhibiting carbonic anhydrase, and can further augment alkalinization.

If alkalinization and hydration are unable to decrease cystine excretion or prevent urolithiasis, or if excretion is greater than 500 mg per day, then cystine-binding therapy should be initiated. The first oral agent ever to be used was D-penicillamine, which binds to cystine and forms a complex that is fifty times more soluble than cystine. Each gram can dissolve 300 mg of cystine. The systemic toxicity of D-penicillamine is responsible for about 50% of patients withdrawing from therapy. Side effects are skin rashes, nausea, loss of taste and smell, fevers, chills, and arthralgia. It also can cause pyridoxine (vitamin B6) deficiency, as D-penicillamine chelates metals; supplementation of pyridoxine may be required.

Thiola (alpha-mercaptopropionylglycine) has a binding action similar to D-penicillamine and has been shown to be as effective in inhibiting renalithiasis. Thiola's major advantage is decreased systemic toxicity. It is now the oral cystine-binding therapy of choice. Oral therapy is initiated at 100 mg three times per day up to a maximum of 800 mg per day. The goal of therapy is to keep the urinary cystine levels less than 250 mg per day. The main side effect to be wary of is oral ulcers. Captopril also binds in a manner comparable to the above agents, and the resulting captopril-cystine complex is 200 times more soluble than cystine itself. It also can decrease urinary cystine levels, and may be the ideal agent in hypertensive patients with cystinuria.

Cystine stones are amenable to irrigation chemolytic therapy, which creates a highly alkaline environment for dissolving cystine. Irrigants, such as N-acetylcysteine (which complexes with cystine) and tromethamine E (which has a pH of 10.6), can be infused via ureteral catheters or nephrostomy tubes. Large and obstructing stones require extracorporeal shock wave lithotripsy (ESWL) and other fragmentation techniques. It has been hypothesized that there may be different crystal structures (rough and smooth forms) of cystine that may explain the inconsistent results of ESWL. Rough cystine is composed of large, organized hexagonal crystals with good cleavage planes; smooth calculi are formed of smaller, disorganized, poorly formed crystals. The upper size limit for ESWL is about 1 cm. Recalcitrant stones may require percutaneous extraction or nephrolithotomy. Frequently, multiple percutaneous procedures for ureteroscopic manipulation are necessary.

In the present patient, the diagnosis was made by observation of hexagonal cystine crystals on a fresh, first morning urine specimen. She elected to undergo ESWL, but the attempt was unsuccessful. She then underwent a successful left percutaneous nephrolithotomy procedure to remove the cystine stones.

Clinical Pearls

1. Cystine stones account for 1–2% of all urinary calculi.

2. Cystinuria is an autosomal recessive disorder of transmembrane transport of dibasic amino acids that results in defective absorption of cystine in the intestine and resorption in the proximal tubule.

3. Hexagonal cystine crystals can be identified on fresh, first morning voided urine specimens.

4. When alkalinizing urine, aim for a urinary pH of 7.5 to maximize solubility of cystine.

5. The goal of therapy is to lower cystine concentration in the urine to less than 200 mg/L.

6. Thiola is the cystine-binding agent of choice. It may be used judiciously in conjunction with hydration and alkalinization of urine if these two methods fail or if cystine excretion is greater than 500 mg per day.

REFERENCES

1. Stoller ML, Bolton DM: Urinary stone disease. In Tanagho EA, McAninich JW (eds): Smith's General Urology. Norwalk, CT, Appleton & Lange, 1995, pp 276–304.
2. Jenkins AD: Calculus formation. In Gillenwater JY, Grayhack JT, Howards SS, Duckett JW (eds): Adult and Pediatric Urology, 3rd ed. St. Louis, Mosby, 1996, pp 461–505.
3. Rutchik SD, Resnick MI: Cystine calculi: Diagnosis and management. Urol Clin North Am 24:163–171, 1997.
4. Menon M, Parulkar BG, Drach GW: Urinary lithiasis: Etiology, diagnosis, and medical management. In Walsh PC, Retik AB, Vaughn ED, Wein AJ (eds): Campbell's Urology, 7th ed. Philadelphia, W.B. Saunders, 1998, pp 2661–2733.

INDEX